A Practical Guide to

# Dermal Filler Procedures

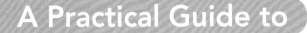
A Practical Guide to

# Dermal Filler Procedures

**Series Editor**

## Rebecca Small, M.D., F.A.A.F.P.

Assistant Clinical Professor,
Family and Community Medicine,
University of California, San Francisco, CA

Director, Medical Aesthetics Training,
Natividad Medical Center,
Family Medicine Residency Program—UCSF Affiliate,
Salinas, CA

**Associate Editor**

## Dalano Hoang, D.C.

Clinic Director,
Monterey Bay Laser Aesthetics,
Capitola, CA

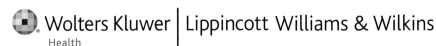
Wolters Kluwer | Lippincott Williams & Wilkins
Health

Philadelphia · Baltimore · New York · London
Buenos Aires · Hong Kong · Sydney · Tokyo

*Acquisitions Editor:* Sonya Seigafuse
*Product Manager:* Kerry Barrett
*Production Manager:* Bridgett Dougherty
*Senior Manufacturing Manager:* Benjamin Rivera
*Marketing Manager:* Kim Schonberger
*Illustrator:* Liana Bauman
*Creative Director:* Doug Smock
*Production Service:* Aptara, Inc.

Printed in China

**Library of Congress Cataloging-in-Publication Data**

Small, Rebecca.
   A practical guide to dermal filler procedures / Rebecca Small ; associate
editor, Dalano Hoang.
      p. ; cm. – (Cosmetic series)
   Includes bibliographical references and index.
   ISBN: 978-1-60913-148-7 (alk. paper)
   I. Hoang, Dalano.   II. Title.   III. Series: Cosmetic series.
   [DNLM: 1. Face–Handbooks.   2. Cosmetic Techniques–Handbooks.   3. Durapatite–
administration & dosage–Handbooks.   4. Hyaluronic Acid–administration &
dosage–Handbooks.   5. Injections, Intradermal–methods–Handbooks.   WE 39]
   LC classification not assigned
   617.5′2059–dc23

                                                                2011032837

Care has been taken to confirm the accuracy of the information presented and to describe generally accepted practices. However, the authors, editors, and publisher are not responsible for errors or omissions or for any consequences from application of the information in this book and make no warranty, expressed or implied, with respect to the currency, completeness, or accuracy of the contents of the publication. Application of the information in a particular situation remains the professional responsibility of the practitioner.

The authors, editors, and publisher have exerted every effort to ensure that drug selection and dosage set forth in this text are in accordance with current recommendations and practice at the time of publication. However, in view of ongoing research, changes in government regulations, and the constant flow of information relating to drug therapy and drug reactions, the reader is urged to check the package insert for each drug for any change in indications and dosage and for added warnings and precautions. This is particularly important when the recommended agent is a new or infrequently employed drug.

Some drugs and medical devices presented in the publication have Food and Drug Administration (FDA) clearance for limited use in restricted research settings. It is the responsibility of the health care providers to ascertain the FDA status of each drug or device planned for use in their clinical practice.

CCS0618

As a lecturer, editor, author, and medical reviewer, I have had ample opportunity to evaluate many speakers as well as extensive medical literature. After reviewing this series of books on cosmetic procedures by Rebecca Small, MD, I have concluded that it has to be one of the best and most detailed, yet practical presentation of the topics that I have ever encountered. As a physician whose practice is limited solely to providing office procedures, I see great value in these texts for clinicians and the patients they serve.

The goal of medical care is to make patients feel better and to help them experience an improved quality of life that extends for an optimal, productive period. Interventions may be directed at the emotional/psychiatric, medical/physical, or self-image areas.

For many physicians, performing medical procedures provides excitement in the practice of medicine. The ability to see what has been accomplished in a concrete way provides the positive feedback we all seek in providing care. Sometimes, it involves removing a tumor. At other times, it may be performing a screening procedure to be sure no disease is present. Maybe it is making patients feel better about their appearance. For whatever reason, the "hands on" practice of medicine is more rewarding for some practitioners.

In the late 1980s and early 1990s, there was resurgence in the interest of performing procedures in primary care. It did not involve hospital procedures but rather those that could be performed in the office. Coincidentally, patients also became interested in less invasive procedures such as laparoscopic cholecystectomy, endometrial ablation, and more. The desire for plastic surgery "extreme makeovers" waned, as technology was developed to provide a gentle, more kind approach to "rejuvenation." Baby boomers were increasing in numbers and wanted to maintain their youthful appearance. This not only improved self-image but it also helped when competing with a younger generation both socially and in the workplace.

These forces then of technological advances, provider interest, and patient desires have led to a huge increase in and demand for "minimally invasive procedures" that has extended to all of medicine. Plastic surgery and aesthetic procedures have indeed been affected by this movement. There have been many new procedures developed in just the last 10–15 years along with constant updates and improvements. As patient demand has soared for these new treatments, physicians have found that there is a whole new world of procedures they need to incorporate into their practice if they are going to provide the latest in aesthetic services.

Rebecca Small, MD, the editor and author of this series of books on cosmetic procedures, has been at the forefront of the aesthetic procedures movement. She has written extensively and conducted numerous workshops to help others learn the latest techniques. She has the practical experience to know just what the physician needs to develop a practice and provides "the latest and the best" in these books. Using her knowledge of the field, she has selected the topics wisely to include

- A Practical Guide to: Botulinum Toxin Procedures
- A Practical Guide to: Dermal Filler Procedures
- A Practical Guide to: Chemical Peels and Skin Care Products
- A Practical Guide to: Cosmetic Laser Procedures

Dr. Small does not just provide a cursory, quick review of these subjects. Rather, they are an in-depth practical guide to performing these procedures. The emphasis here should be on "practical" and "in-depth." There is no extra esoteric waste of words, yet every procedure is explained in a clear, concise, useful format that allows practitioners of all levels of experience to learn and gain from reading these texts.

The basic outline of these books consists of the pertinent anatomy, the specific indications and contraindications, specific how-to diagrams and explanations on performing the procedures, complications and how to deal with them, tables with comparisons and amounts of materials needed, before and after patient instructions as well as consent forms (an immense time-saving feature), sample procedure notes, and a list of supply sources. An extensive updated bibliography is provided in each text for further reading. Photos are abundant depicting the performance of the procedures as well as before and after results. These comprehensive texts are clearly written for the practitioner who wants to "learn everything" about the topics covered. Patients definitely desire these procedures and Dr. Small has provided the information to meet the physician demand to learn them.

For those interested in aesthetic procedures, these books will be a godsend. Even for those not so interested in performing the procedures described, the reading is easy and interesting and will update the readers on what is currently available so that they might better advise their patients.

Dr. Small has truly written a one-of-a-kind series of books on Cosmetic Procedures. It is my prediction that it will be received very well and be most appreciated by all who make use of it.

*John L. Pfenninger, M.D., F.A.A.F.P.*
*Founder and President, The Medical Procedures Center*
*PC Founder and Senior Consultant, The National Procedures Institute*
*Clinical Professor of Family Medicine, Michigan State College*
*of Human Medicine*

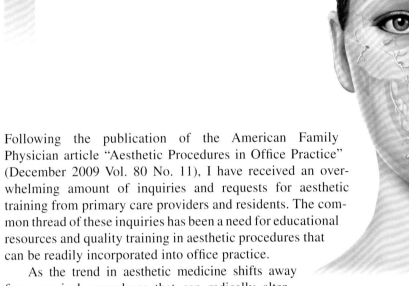

Following the publication of the American Family Physician article "Aesthetic Procedures in Office Practice" (December 2009 Vol. 80 No. 11), I have received an overwhelming amount of inquiries and requests for aesthetic training from primary care providers and residents. The common thread of these inquiries has been a need for educational resources and quality training in aesthetic procedures that can be readily incorporated into office practice.

As the trend in aesthetic medicine shifts away from surgical procedures that can radically alter appearance, toward procedures that have minimal recovery time and offer more subtle enhancements, the number of minimally invasive aesthetic procedures performed continues to increase. These procedures, which include dermal filler and botulinum toxin injections, lasers and light-based technologies, and chemical peels, have become the primary modalities for treatment of facial aging and skin rejuvenation. This aesthetic procedure series is designed to be a truly practical guide for primary care physicians, physician assistants, nurse practitioners, residents in training, and other healthcare providers interested in aesthetics. It is not comprehensive but is inclusive of current minimally invasive aesthetic procedures that can be readily incorporated into office practice to directly benefit our patients.

The goal of this dermal filler injection book, the second in the aesthetic practical guide series, is to provide a step-by-step approach to dermal filler treatments. The introduction serves as a foundation and provides basic aesthetic medicine concepts essential to successfully performing aesthetic procedures. Each chapter is dedicated to a single dermal filler procedure with all relevant anatomy reviewed, including the target regions as well as areas to be avoided. There is an accompanying website with videos demonstrating each procedure. Injection sites are highlighted to help providers perform procedures more effectively and minimize complication risks. Recommended anesthesia methods, an integral part of dermal filler treatments, are included for each procedure along with suggestions for management of the most commonly encountered issues seen in follow-up visits. More experienced injectors may appreciate the concise summary of each procedure's complications and up-to-date suggestions for management, advanced treatment techniques, combining aesthetic treatments to maximize outcomes, current product developments and reimbursement recommendations.

When getting started, providers are encouraged to begin with the basic dermal filler procedures for treatment of nasolabial folds, marionette lines and mental crease, and progress to advanced procedures as skill is acquired. Basic procedures utilize straightforward injection techniques and products which are more moldable and forgiving. They typically achieve good outcomes, have a low incidence of side effects, and are associated with high patient satisfaction. Advanced dermal filler procedures such as facial sculpting and contouring, can be used for treatment of more complex aging changes and for enhancement purposes. Longer lasting products along with more challenging injection techniques are required with advanced procedures.

This book is intended to serve as a guide and not a replacement for experience. When learning aesthetic procedural skills, a formal training course is recommended, as well as preceptorship with a skilled provider.

# Acknowledgments

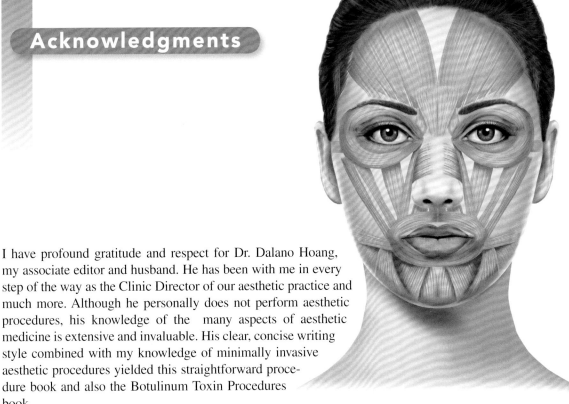

I have profound gratitude and respect for Dr. Dalano Hoang, my associate editor and husband. He has been with me in every step of the way as the Clinic Director of our aesthetic practice and much more. Although he personally does not perform aesthetic procedures, his knowledge of the many aspects of aesthetic medicine is extensive and invaluable. His clear, concise writing style combined with my knowledge of minimally invasive aesthetic procedures yielded this straightforward procedure book and also the Botulinum Toxin Procedures book.

A special thanks to Dr. John L. Pfenninger and Dr. E.J. Mayeaux who have inspired and supported me, and taught me much about educating and writing.

The University of California, San Francisco, and the Natividad Medical Center family medicine residents deserve special recognition. Their interest and enthusiasm for aesthetic procedures led me to develop the first family medicine aesthetics training curriculum in 2008. Special recognition is also due to the primary care providers who participated in my aesthetic courses at the American Academy of Family Physicians national conferences over the years. Their questions and input further solidified the need for this practical guide series.

I am indebted to my Capitola office staff for their ongoing logistical and administrative support which made it possible to write this series.

Special acknowledgments are due to those at Wolters Kluwer Health who made this book series possible, in particular, Kerry Barrett, Sonya Seigafuse, Freddie Patane, Brett MacNaughton, and Doug Smock. It has been a pleasure working with Liana Bauman, the gifted artist who created all of the illustrations for these books.

Finally, I dedicate this second book in the series also to my 5-year-old son, Kaidan Hoang, for the unending hugs and kisses that greeted me no matter how late I got home from working on this project.

# Contents

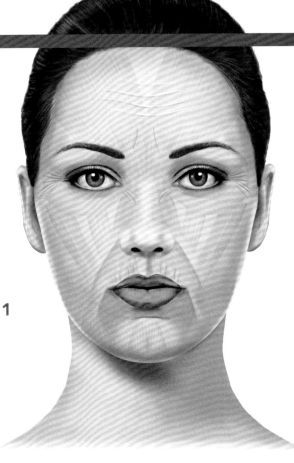

 *A video clip for every procedure can be found on the book's website.*

# Dermal Filler Anatomy

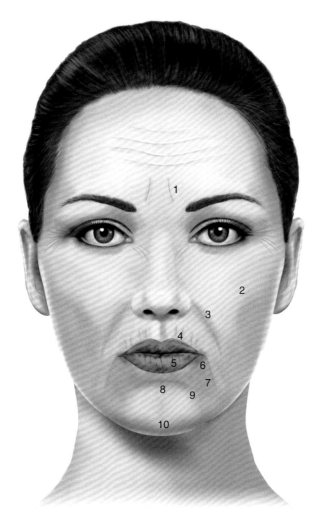

1. Frown lines
   (Glabellar rhytids)
2. Cheek flattening
   (Malar atropy)
3. Nasolabial folds
   (Melolabial folds)
4. Lip lines
   (Perioral rhytids)
5. Lip thinning
   (Lip atrophy)
6. Downturned corners of mouth
   (Depressed oral commissures)
7. Marionette lines
   (Melomental folds)
8. Chin line or mental crease
   (Labiomental crease)
9. Extended mental crease
   (Extended labiomental crease)
10. Chin flattening
    (Mentum atrophy)

*FIGURE 1* ● Wrinkles, folds, and contour irregularities of the face—anterior-posterior (medical term).

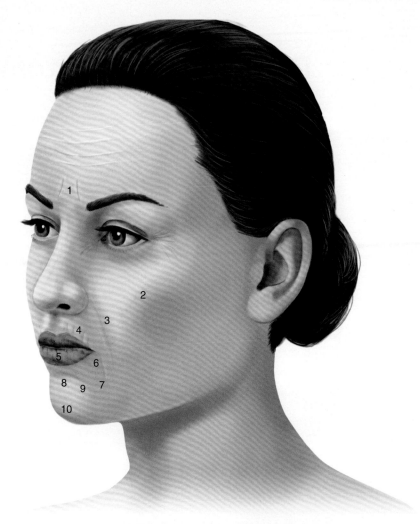

1. Frown lines
   (Glabellar rhytids)
2. Cheek flattening
   (Malar atrophy)
3. Nasolabial folds
   (Melolabial atrophy)
4. Lip lines
   (Perioral rhytids)
5. Lip thinning
   (Lip atrophy)
6. Downturned corners of mouth
   (Depressed oral commissures)
7. Marionette lines
   (Melomental folds)
8. Chin line or mental crease
   (Labiomental crease)
9. Extended mental crease
   (Extended labiomental crease)
10. Chin flattening
    (Mentum atrophy)

*FIGURE 2* ● Wrinkles, folds, and contour irregularities of the face—oblique (medical term).

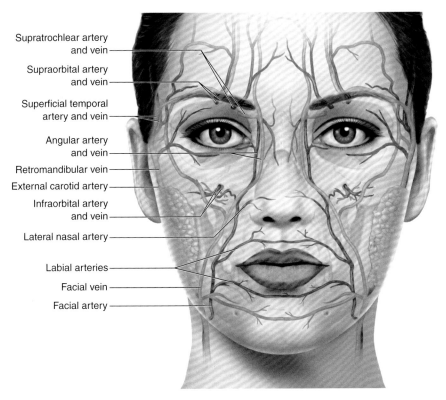

Supratrochlear artery and vein

Supraorbital artery and vein

Superficial temporal artery and vein

Angular artery and vein

Retromandibular vein

External carotid artery

Infraorbital artery and vein

Lateral nasal artery

Labial arteries

Facial vein

Facial artery

**FIGURE 3** ● Vascular supply of the face.

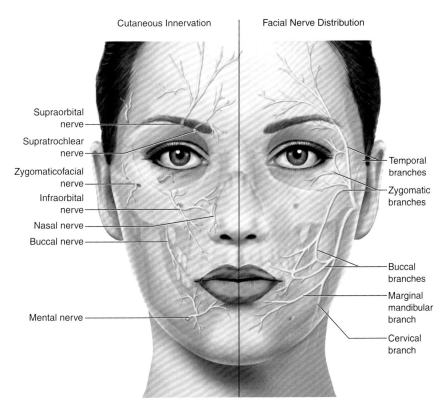

Cutaneous Innervation

Facial Nerve Distribution

Supraorbital nerve

Supratrochlear nerve

Zygomaticofacial nerve

Infraorbital nerve

Nasal nerve

Buccal nerve

Mental nerve

Temporal branches

Zygomatic branches

Buccal branches

Marginal mandibular branch

Cervical branch

**FIGURE 4** ● Nerves of the face.

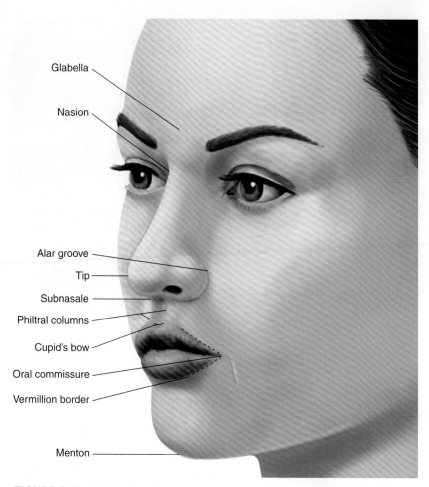

Glabella

Nasion

Alar groove

Tip

Subnasale

Philtral columns

Cupid's bow

Oral commissure

Vermillion border

Menton

*FIGURE 5* ● Facial landmarks.

# Introduction and Foundation Concepts

Rebecca Small, M.D.

Dermal filler treatments have become one of the most commonly performed cosmetic procedures in the United States, second only to botulinum toxin treatments, according to statistics from the American Society for Aesthetic Plastic Surgery. They have advanced beyond their primary indication as treatment for facial wrinkles and folds to more sophisticated applications of facial sculpting and contouring. Dermal Fillers are a versatile and elegant tool for facial rejuvenation and filler injection is an essential skill for physicians and qualified healthcare providers who wish to incorporate aesthetic medicine into their practice.

Currently available fillers vary in composition, duration of action, palpability, administration techniques, complications, and other factors. Achieving desirable outcomes and minimizing the risk of complications depend equally on the provider's injection skills, knowledge of dermal filler products and anatomy, as well as an appreciation for aesthetic facial proportions and symmetry.

## Facial Aging

Facial aging is associated with a gradual thinning of the skin and loss of elasticity over time accompanied by diminishment of dermal collagen, hyaluronic acid (HA), and elastin. This intrinsic aging process is accelerated and compounded by sun damage and other extrinsic factors such as smoking, resulting in facial lines and wrinkles (also called rhytids or rhytides). Habitual muscle contraction with facial expression also contributes to formation of wrinkles, particularly in the upper one-third of the face. These dynamic wrinkles are typically treated with botulinum toxin injections. In the lower two-thirds of the face volume loss and laxity are more evident and dermal fillers are most commonly used in this region (Figs. 1 and 2). Lines and wrinkles in this area are typically visible when the face is at rest, which are referred to as static lines. Facial volume loss, also referred to as biometric reduction, results from resorption of facial bones, degradation of subcutaneous tissue, and descent of the fat pads. Facial contours change with age from high cheeks and a small chin (Fig. 3A) to a bottom-heavy appearance with flattened cheeks and prominent jowls (Fig. 3B).

## Basic and Advanced Procedures

The treatment area, type of product (temporary, semipermanent, permanent, etc.), and injection techniques used determine the level of complexity for dermal filler procedures. When getting started with dermal filler injection, it is advisable to start with the basic dermal filler procedures described below, acquire proficiency, and then proceed to the advanced procedures.

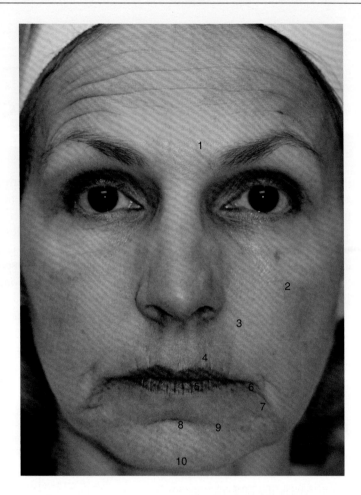

1. Frown lines
   (Glabellar rhytids)
2. Cheek flattening
   (Malar atrophy)
3. Nasolabial folds
   (Melolabial folds)
4. Lip lines
   (Perioral rhytids)
5. Lip thinning
   (Lip atrophy)

6. Downturned corners of mouth
   (Depressed oral commissures)
7. Marionette lines
   (Melomental folds)
8. Chin line or mental crease
   (Labiomental crease)
9. Extended mental crease
   (Extended labiomental crease)
10. Chin flattening
    (Mentum atrophy)

*FIGURE 1* ● Facial wrinkles, folds, and contour irregularities-anterior-posterior (medical term).

## Basic Procedures

Recommended dermal filler products for basic procedures include Prevelle Silk®, Juvederm®, and Restylane® all of which are hyaluronic acids (HAs). These dermal fillers are generally easier to handle, with good flow characteristics during injection in tissue, requiring gentle plunger pressure. Once injected, they feel supple and are easily molded and compressed, which reduces the risk of undesired product collections and contour irregularities. In addition, HA products can be degraded using injectable hyaluronidase for correction if necessary. Treatment areas for basic procedures are listed in Table 1.

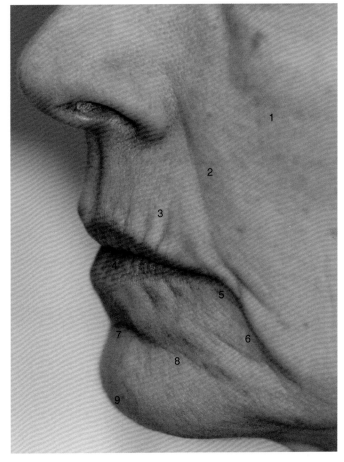

1. Cheek flattening
   (Malar atrophy)
2. Nasolabial folds
   (Melolabial folds)
3. Lip lines
   (Perioral rhytids)
4. Lip thinning
   (Lip atrophy)
5. Downturned corners of mouth
   (Depressed oral commissures)
6. Marionette lines
   (Melomental folds)
7. Chin line or mental crease
   (Labiomental crease)
8. Extended mental crease
   (Extended labiomental crease)
9. Chin flattening
   (Mentum atrophy)

**FIGURE 2** ● Facial wrinkles, folds and contour irregularities-lateral (medical term).

Dermal filler treatments in these facial areas yield predictable results, have the greatest efficacy, fewest side effects, and are preferred for providers getting started with dermal filler procedures. Injection techniques for basic procedures include linear threading, fanning, and cross-hatching (see Techniques for Dermal Filler Injection below).

## Advanced Procedures

Recommended dermal filler products for advanced procedures include the products used for basic procedures as well as Perlane® and Radiesse®. Perlane and Radiesse tend to

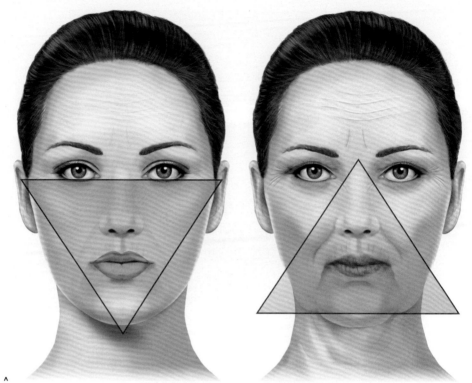

^
*FIGURE 3* ● Facial aging progression from youthful (**A**) to aged (**B**) contours.

have increased longevity compared to the basic dermal fillers. They also offer advantages of significant structural support in tissue and are useful for facial contouring, in addition to soft tissue filling. Greater plunger pressure during treatment and more practiced injection skill are typically necessary with advanced dermal fillers. Treatment areas for advanced procedures are listed in Table 1. Dermal filler treatments in these areas often require precise placement of small volumes and can be associated with greater risks and longer lasting complications. Injection techniques for advanced procedures include those used for basic procedures as well as depot and layering techniques (see Techniques for Dermal Filler Injection below). It is advisable to obtain injection proficiency and confidence with basic dermal filler procedures before proceeding to more advanced procedures.

## Dermal Filler Indications

- The U.S. Food and Drug Administration (FDA) approved the injection of HA and calcium hydroxylapatite (CaHA) dermal fillers into the mid- or deep dermis for correction of moderate to severe facial wrinkles and folds, such as nasolabial folds and marionette lines.
- Radiesse, a CaHA dermal filler, has also been FDA approved for the treatment of HIV-associated facial lipoatrophy.
- Dermal filler treatment of lips and other cosmetic areas are considered off-label.

## TABLE 1

### Basic and Advanced Dermal Filler Treatment Areas

| Dermal Filler Treatment Areas | |
| --- | --- |
| Common Name | Medical Term |
| **Basic** | |
| Nasolabial folds | Melolabial folds |
| Marionette lines and downturned corners of the mouth | Melomental folds and depressed oral commissures |
| Mental crease | Labiomental crease |
| **Advanced** | |
| Frown lines | Glabellar rhytids |
| Cheek flattening | Malar atrophy |
| Lip lines | Perioral rhytids |
| Lip thinning (lip border and body) | Lip atrophy |
| Extended mental crease | Extended labiomental crease |
| Chin flattening | Mentum atrophy |
| Scars | Depression scars |

## Patient Selection

Dermal filler procedures are most commonly performed as corrective measures for patients with skin aging to smooth static lines and wrinkles, particularly in the lower two-thirds of the face, such as nasolabial folds and marionette lines. They are also performed for augmentation purposes and facial contouring, such as lip and malar enhancement. It is important to set the expectation that dermal fillers will soften lines and wrinkles as opposed to erase them, and that subtle improvements in contours can be achieved but fillers do not offer surgery-like results. Patients with excessive skin laxity and folds usually require surgical intervention for significant improvements. Patients with unrealistic expectations or body dysmorphic disorder are not candidates for aesthetic treatments.

## Products

Dermal fillers are categorized on the basis of duration of action: short-acting (less than 4 months), long-acting (6 months to 1 year), semipermanent (1–2 years), and permanent (2 years or more). A historical overview of dermal filler products used in the United States is shown in Figure 4, which highlights the increased duration of action that has been achieved with new product formulations over time. Table 2 lists available dermal filler products in the United Sates that are in common use. According to statistics from the American Society for Aesthetic Plastic Surgery, HA is most frequently used. The focus of this book is HA fillers, along with a longer acting product, CaHA, due to their versatility, safety profiles, and ease of administration.

## TABLE 2

### Dermal Fillers Commonly Used in the United States

| Agent | Component | Company | Duration |
|---|---|---|---|
| **Short-acting** | | | |
| Prevelle Silk® | Hyaluronic acid with lidocaine | Mentor | 2–4 mo |
| **Long-acting** | | | |
| Hydrelle® | Hyaluronic acid with lidocaine | Anika | 6–12 mo |
| Juvederm Ultra®/Juvederm® Ultra XC | Hyaluronic acid without/with lidocaine | Allergan | 6–12 mo |
| Juvederm Ultra Plus®/ Juvederm Ultra Plus® XC | Hyaluronic acid without/with lidocaine | Allergan | 6–12 mo |
| Perlane®/Perlane®-L | Hyaluronic acid without/with lidocaine | Medicis | 6–12 mo |
| Restylane®/Restylane®-L | Hyaluronic acid without/with lidocaine | Medicis | 6–12 mo |
| **Semipermanent** | | | |
| Radiesse® | Calcium hydroxylapatite | Merz | 1–1½ yr |
| Sculptra® | Poly-L-lactic acid | Dermik | 1–2 yr |
| **Permanent** | | | |
| ArteFill® | Polymethyl methacrylate with bovine collagen | Artes | Permanent |

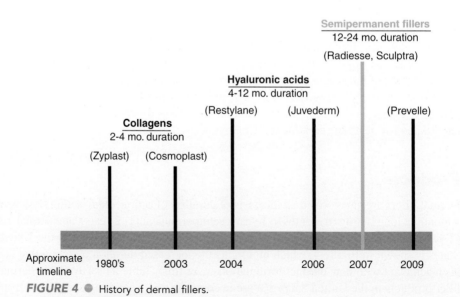

FIGURE 4 ● History of dermal fillers.

HA is a naturally occurring glycosaminoglycan in the dermal extracellular matrix that provides structural support and nutrients and, through its hydrophilic capacity, adds volume and fullness to the skin. Commercially available HAs vary in formulation, concentration, and degree of cross-linkage which affects their duration of action as well as postprocedure risks of swelling. For example, Juvederm Ultra has 24 mg/mL of HA and typically has mild to moderate postprocedure swelling, compared with Hydrelle, which has 28 mg/mL of HA, and can be associated with more significant postprocedure swelling. HA formulation also affects tissue filling effects. Some HA products have softer tissue filling effects such as Juvederm Ultra XC, whereas others have firmer tissue filling effects such as Juvederm Ultra Plus XC and Restylane-L.

HA products are clear, colorless gels (Fig. 5). Some HAs are formulated with lidocaine (referred to as HA-lidocaine in this book) to increase patient comfort during injection and reduce the need for anesthesia. Maximum treatment doses of HA dermal filler vary by manufacturer and are reported in the product package insert. For example, the maximum dose for Juvederm is 20 mL per year and for Restylane is 6.0 mL per patient per treatment.

Radiesse, the currently available CaHA filler, consists of CaHA microspheres (30%) suspended in a carboxymethylcellulose gel (70%). After CaHA injection, the gel is absorbed at approximately 3 months, at which time the patient's native fibroblasts are stimulated to synthesize new collagen. CaHA offers significant structural support to tissues into which it is injected. CaHA is a white opaque product (Fig. 5). CaHA has also been FDA approved to be mixed with small amounts of lidocaine, which reduces product viscosity and provides some anesthesia.

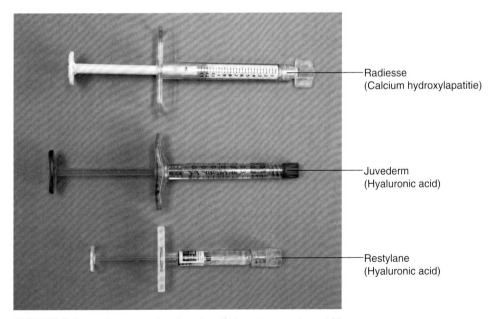

Radiesse
(Calcium hydroxylapatitie)

Juvederm
(Hyaluronic acid)

Restylane
(Hyaluronic acid)

*FIGURE 5* ● Hyaluronic acid and calcium hydroxylapatite dermal fillers.

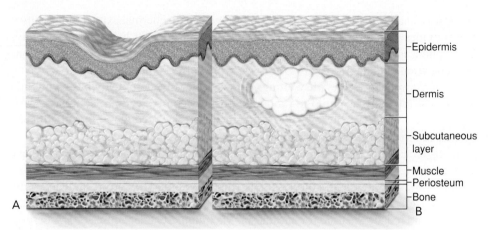

A                                                                                        B

*FIGURE 6* ● Mechanism of action for dermal fillers.

## Mechanism of Action

Dermal fillers correct wrinkles and augment facial contours by filling a volume deficit either in the dermis or in deeper tissue spaces. This process is shown in Figure 6 in which a volume deficit representing either a skin wrinkle (e.g., frown line) or contour defect (e.g., malar flattening) (Fig. 6A) is smoothed after dermal filler injection (Fig. 6B).

Dermal fillers can also be categorized according to their mechanism of action into space-occupying fillers and biostimulants. Space-occupying fillers replace lost volume without effecting significant change in adjacent tissues, whereas biostimulants stimulate fibroblasts to synthesize new collagen. Common space-occupying dermal fillers include collagen and HA; common biostimulants include CaHA and poly-L-lactic acid.

## Product Selection

Dermal filler selection at the time of treatment is dependent on several factors. The treatment area and the severity of volume loss are considered initially. Certain areas such as lips, scars, and frown lines require a thinner, more supple filler, whereas a more structural filler is required for other areas such as the chin and malars. Superficial lines require more supple fillers whereas deep volume loss is treated with more structural fillers. Longevity of results is also an important consideration. Collagen products typically last 4 months or less, HAs 4–12 months, and CaHA 12–18 months. Providers' knowledge and experience with available types of dermal fillers also contribute to product selection.

## Calcium Hydroxylapatite and Lidocaine Preparation

CaHA may be used directly from the syringe or may be mixed with small amounts of lidocaine to reduce viscosity. For certain dermal filler treatments that benefit from more structural support, such as chin augmentation, it is not recommended to mix CaHA with lidocaine. For most treatments with CaHA, however, preparation with lidocaine can provide additional patient comfort and ease of injection. The mixing procedure for

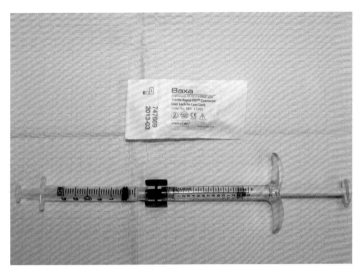

FIGURE 7 ● Calcium hydroxylapatite mixing with lidocaine.

preparing CaHA with lidocaine (CaHA-lidocaine) is described below using Radiesse. Treatments using CaHA with lidocaine in this book include the extended mental crease, perioral lip lines, malar augmentation, and layering for deep volume loss of nasolabial folds, marionette lines, and the mental crease.

CaHA-lidocaine preparation procedure:

1. Uncap the 1.5-mL Radiesse syringe and attach a luer-to-luer connector.
2. Prime the connector by gently pushing the Radiesse plunger until the connector is filled with dermal filler product.
3. Using a 3.0-mL syringe and an 18-gauge, 1½-inch needle, draw up 0.3 mL of lidocaine HCl 2% with epinephrine 1:100,000.
4. Connect to the luer-to-luer connector, which is attached to the Radiesse syringe, to the 3.0-mL syringe. The connector should be between the Radiesse and the 3.0-mL syringes (Fig. 7).
5. Gently push all contents from the Radiesse syringe into the 3.0-mL syringe and then back into the Radiesse syringe. Mix slowly to avoid the formation of bubbles in the product. Repeat this process approximately 10 times until the mixture is uniform.
6. Disconnect the luer-to-luer connector from the Radiesse syringe and attach the applicable needle for treatment.
7. Save the 3.0-mL syringe. It will contain residual Radiesse, which can be added to the Radiesse syringe and used for treatment.

## Alternative Therapies

Other available treatments of facial lines and wrinkles include botulinum toxin for dynamic wrinkles, skin resurfacing procedures such as microdermabrasion, chemical peels, and nonablative or ablative laser treatments of static lines. For severe wrinkling with sagging lax skin, surgical treatment such as a facelift is an option. Facial contouring of the malar and chin areas can also be achieved surgically with permanent implants.

## Contraindications

- Pregnancy or nursing
- Infection in the treatment area (e.g., herpes simplex, acne)
- Hypertrophic or keloidal scar formation
- Bleeding abnormality (e.g., thrombocytopenia, anticoagulant use)
- Accutane use within the last 6 months
- Skin atrophy (e.g., chronic steroid use, genetic syndromes such as Ehlers-Danlos syndrome)
- Impaired healing (e.g., due to immunosuppression)
- Dermatoses active in the treatment area (e.g., vitiligo, psoriasis, eczema)
- Uncontrolled systemic condition
- Previous anaphylactic reaction
- Multiple severe allergies
- Sensitivity or allergy to constituents of dermal filler products
- Body dysmorphic disorder
- Unrealistic expectations

## Advantages of Dermal Fillers

- Immediately visible results
- With temporary fillers, most undesirable outcomes spontaneously resolve

## Disadvantages of Dermal Filler

- Temporary swelling and bruising posttreatment can occur.
- Repeat treatments are necessary to maintain results.

## Equipment

- General
  - Gloves nonsterile
  - Alcohol pads
  - Gauze 3 × 3 inches, nonwoven
  - Wooden cotton-tipped applicators
  - Surgical marker or soft, white eyeliner pencil for marking the treatment area
  - Handheld mirror
- Anesthesia
  - 1.0-mL, 3.0-mL, and 5.0-mL Luer-Lok™ tip syringes
  - Lidocaine HCl 2% with epinephrine 1:100,000
  - Lidocaine HCl 2% without epinephrine
  - Sodium bicarbonate 8.4%
  - 18-gauge, 1½-inch needle (to draw up)
  - 30-gauge, ½-inch needle (for injection)
  - Topical benzocaine 20% (CaineTips™ or gel)
  - BLT ointment (benzocaine 20%: lidocaine 6%: tetracaine 4%)
  - Ethyl chloride mist spray
  - Ice or contact cooling device (e.g., ArTek Spot®)

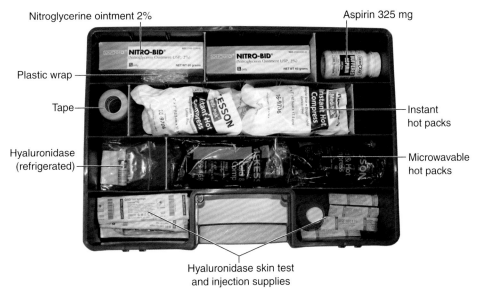

Nitroglycerine ointment 2%

Aspirin 325 mg

Plastic wrap

Tape

Instant hot packs

Hyaluronidase (refrigerated)

Microwavable hot packs

Hyaluronidase skin test and injection supplies

FIGURE 8 ● Emergency vascular occlusion kit.

- CaHA (Radiesse) mixing with lidocaine
  - 1.5-mL Radiesse prefilled syringe
  - 0.3 mL of lidocaine HCl 2% with epinephrine 1:100,000
  - 3.0-mL Luer-Lok tip syringe (supplied with Radiesse)
  - Luer-to-luer connector (supplied with Radiesse)
- Dermal filler procedure
  - Dermal filler prefilled syringes
  - 30-gauge, ½-inch needles (for Juvederm and Restylane)
  - 27-gauge, 1¼-inch needles (for Radiesse)
  - 28-gauge, ¾-inch needle (for Radiesse, supplied with Radiesse)
- Emergency vascular occlusion kit (Fig. 8)
  - Hot packs
  - Hyaluronidase (150 units/mL)
  - 1.0-mL Luer-Lok tip syringe
  - 18-gauge, 1½-inch needles (for drawing up hyaluronidase)
  - 30-gauge, ½-inch needles (for injecting)
  - Aspirin 325 mg, chewable
  - Nitroglycerine ointment 2%
  - Plastic wrap (for occluding nitroglycerin)

## Handling

HA dermal fillers are supplied in individual prepackaged syringes ranging from 0.4 to 1.0 mL, based on the manufacturer. CaHA dermal fillers are supplied as 0.3-, 0.8-, and 1.5-mL prepackaged syringes and include supplies for mixing with lidocaine. Syringes are typically stored at room temperature (up to 25°C or 77°F) prior to use. Product shelf life is usually 1–2 years. HA dermal fillers formulated with lidocaine have a shorter shelf life. The specific manufacturer package insert guidelines should be followed for storage and handling.

## Anatomy

- Wrinkles, folds, and contour irregularities of the face—anterior-posterior (see Dermal Filler Anatomy section, Fig. 1)
- Wrinkles, folds, and contour irregularities of the face—oblique (see Dermal Filler Anatomy section, Fig. 3)
- Vascular supply of the face (see Dermal Filler Anatomy section, Fig. 4)
- Nerves of the face (see Dermal Filler Anatomy section, Fig. 5)
- Facial landmarks (see Dermal Filler Anatomy section, Fig. 6)

## Aesthetic Consultation

Understanding the patient's goals and priorities for treatment and setting realistic expectations for results are essential to achieving high levels of patient satisfaction and desired outcomes. This is accomplished with a thorough history and physical examination and formulation of an individualized aesthetic treatment plan as described below.

Review the patient's complete medical history including medications, allergies, and conditions contraindicating treatment; cosmetic history including minimally invasive procedures and plastic surgeries as well as any side effects and satisfaction with results; and social history including upcoming events. A sample patient intake form is shown in Appendix 1, Aesthetic Intake Form. Patients with unrealistic expectations or body dysmorphic disorder often present with a history of repeated dissatisfaction with prior aesthetic treatments. Examine the areas of concern with the patient holding a mirror and have the patient prioritize the treatment areas. Document any asymmetries or unusual findings in the chart.

Educate the patient about the nature of his or her aesthetic issues and discuss treatment options and alternatives. Early in the consultation process, assess whether the patient will benefit most from surgical intervention or minimally invasive treatments. Formulate an individualized aesthetic treatment plan based on the patient's concerns and observed facial aging changes. Review details of the proposed dermal filler and associated anesthesia for the procedure, realistic expectations for results, typical recovery time, anticipated dermal filler volume necessary for treatment, and procedure cost.

Risks of side effects and complications associated with the proposed procedure and anesthesia are discussed, allowing ample opportunity for all questions to be asked and answered. Patients seeking elective aesthetic treatments typically have high expectations for treatment results and low tolerance for side effects and complications. In addition to having a consent form signed by the patient, it is also important to document the informed consent discussion. A sample consent form for dermal filler treatments is shown in Appendix 3, Consent for Dermal Filler Treatments Form.

Photodocumentation is an important part of aesthetic procedures and involves the use of photographs to demonstrate findings at baseline and results after treatments. Consent for photographs is typically included in the procedure consent form. The usual patient positions for photographs include head fully upright looking straight ahead, 45 degrees and 90 degrees. Photographs are taken of the full face and specific treatment areas with the face at rest and with active facial movements.

# Preprocedure Checklist

- Perform an aesthetic consultation and obtain informed consent as described above, including discussion and documentation of the risks, benefits, and complications associated with the procedure and anesthesia, alternatives to the intended procedure, and place the signed consent forms in the chart.
- Take pretreatment photographs with the patient at rest and actively contracting the muscles in the intended treatment area.
- Document and discuss any notable asymmetries or findings prior to the treatment.
- Discuss the type of dermal filler product(s) to be used, estimated volume necessary for the treatment, and cost with the patient prior to the treatment.
- Instruct the patient to avoid aspirin (any product containing acetylsalicylic acid), vitamin E, St. John's wort, and other dietary supplements including ginkgo, evening primrose oil, garlic, feverfew, ginseng, or other herbs and supplements that have anticoagulation properties for 2 weeks prior to the treatment.
- Instruct the patient to discontinue other nonsteroidal anti-inflammatory medications and alcohol consumption 2 days prior to the treatment.
- Provide prophylactic antiviral medication for a history of labial or facial herpes simplex or herpes zoster (e.g., valacyclovir 500 mg, one tablet twice daily) 2 days prior to the procedure and continue for 3 days postprocedure.

# Anesthesia

Providing adequate anesthesia is essential to successfully performing dermal filler procedures. Anesthesia is ideally accomplished with minimal tissue distortion of the treatment area to preserve the baseline anatomy. The main methods for providing anesthesia with dermal filler treatments are reviewed in the Anesthesia section.

# Dermal Filler Injection

## General Injection Principles

- For dermal filler treatments, the needle entry point, also called the injection point or insertion point, is identified by laying the needle against the skin over the treatment area. The length of the needle should correspond to the desired treatment area and the injection point is located at the needle hub (Figs. 9A and 9B).
- Dermal fillers are injected using firm, constant pressure on the syringe plunger. Plunger pressure is released just before pulling the needle out of the skin to avoid tracking dermal filler product in the epidermis.
- Dermal filler is injected confluently and evenly in the treatment area. Achieving smooth dermal filler placement, in the appropriate level of the skin, is an acquired skill for the injector.
- If injecting at the incorrect level, withdraw the needle to the skin insertion and retry.
- After injection, the treatment area is palpated to assess for confluent placement of filler and smoothness. If skipped areas are palpable, additional filler is used to fill these skipped areas.
- If dermal filler is visibly or palpably bumpy, smoothing is required. Filler bumps can usually be smoothed by compressing the product using the following methods:
  - **Two fingers.** Place one finger intraorally and one extraorally to compress the product between the two fingers (Fig. 10).

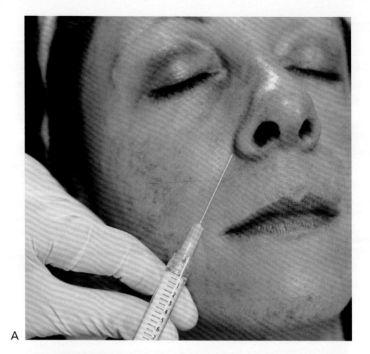

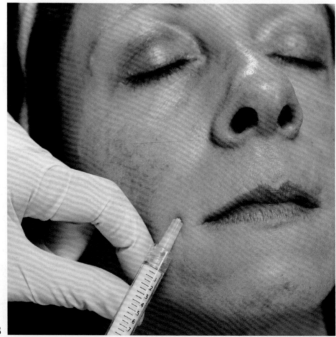

*FIGURE 9* ● Injection points are determined by laying the needle over the treatment area **(A)** and the insertion point is at the needle hub **(B)**.

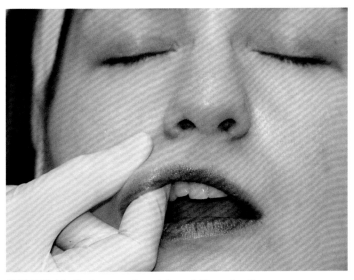

*FIGURE 10* ● Compression of dermal filler using fingers.

- **Cotton-tipped applicator.** Use one finger intraorally and rolling a cotton-tipped applicator with firm pressure slowly over the bump (Fig. 11).
- **Against bone.** Use fingertips or thumbs extraorally to compress the product firmly against the underlying bone (Fig. 12).
- Achieve desired results in one area before beginning injection in another treatment area.
- Needles may become obstructed with Radiesse, particularly with supraperiosteal depot injections. If plunger resistance is encountered while injecting Radiesse, the needle is

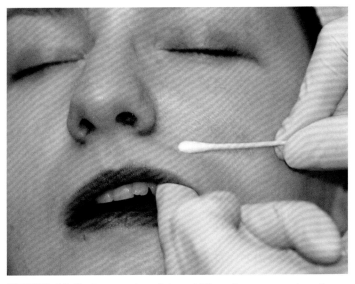

*FIGURE 11* ● Compression of dermal filler using a cotton-tipped applicator.

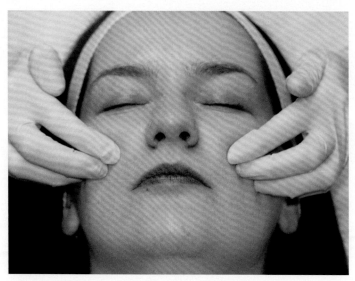

*FIGURE 12* ● Compression of dermal filler against bone.

likely obstructed. Withdraw the needle from the skin and prime it by depressing the plunger to observe for extrusion of product from the needle tip. If no product is extruded, place a new needle on the Radiesse syringe, prime the needle, and resume injection.

### Tip

- Tissue ischemia can result from vascular compromise due to intravascular injection or overfilling tissues with dermal filler. If this occurs, discontinue injection, massage the area until the tissue appears pink, and institute other measures outlined in the Complications section.

### Depth of Injection

Dermal fillers can be injected at different tissue depths, from the deep supraperiosteal plane to the superficial dermis (Fig. 13). Basic dermal filler treatments primarily involve injection in the mid- to deep dermis, whereas more advanced treatments range in depths. For example, the advanced technique of layering involves placing more robust structural dermal filler products, such as CaHA, in the mid- to deep dermis and placing thinner products, such as HAs, in the overlying superficial dermis. Advanced facial contour correction, such as malar augmentation, involves supraperiosteal placement.

The depth of injection can be determined by several factors such as the feel of the needle moving through tissue, plunger resistance during injection, and visibility of the needle tip in the skin. Table 3 lists specific characteristics for different injection depths. It is important to note that if the gray tip of the needle is visible in the skin, injection is too superficial and the needle should be withdrawn and redirected to a deeper level in the skin.

## Techniques for Dermal Filler Injection

- **Linear thread.** The fundamental injection technique for placing dermal filler in tissue is the retrograde linear thread. Insert the needle at the desired tissue depth and

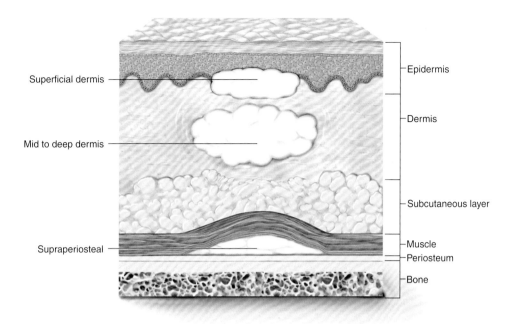

Superficial dermis

Mid to deep dermis

Supraperiosteal

Epidermis

Dermis

Subcutaneous layer

Muscle
Periosteum

Bone

*FIGURE 13* ● Injection depths of dermal fillers.

## TABLE 3

### Injection Depth Characteristics

| Skin Depth | Injection Characteristics |
|---|---|
| Superficial dermis | • Significant resistance when advancing the needle<br>• Significant resistance during injection<br>• Gray needle may be visible in the skin *if injection is too superficial* |
| Mid- to deep dermis | • Some resistance as needle advances through the tissue<br>• Some plunger resistance during injection<br>• Needle tip is not visible |
| Subcutaneous layer | • Minimal to no resistance when advancing the needle<br>• Minimal to no resistance during injection<br>• Needle tip is not visible |
| Supraperiosteal | • Crunchiness as the needle advances through the muscle and a tap on the bone<br>• Minimal to no resistance during injection<br>• Needle tip is deeply placed in tissues and not visible |

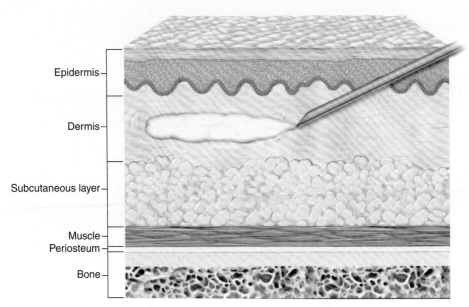

Epidermis

Dermis

Subcutaneous layer

Muscle
Periosteum

Bone

**FIGURE 14** ● Linear threading injection technique with dermal fillers.

depress the plunger firmly as the needle is smoothly withdrawn (Fig. 14). Release the plunger pressure just before pulling the needle out of the skin to avoid tracking dermal filler product in the epidermis.

- **Fanning.** A single needle insertion point is used to inject a series of adjacent linear threads placing dermal filler product in a triangular area. Insert the needle at the desired tissue depth, advance the needle to the hub, and inject filler in a linear thread as the needle is slowly withdrawn; without fully withdrawing the needle from the skin, redirect the needle using small angulations, advance needle to the hub again and repeat until desired correction is achieved (Fig. 15).

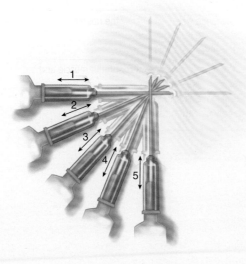

**FIGURE 15** ● Fanning injection technique with dermal fillers.

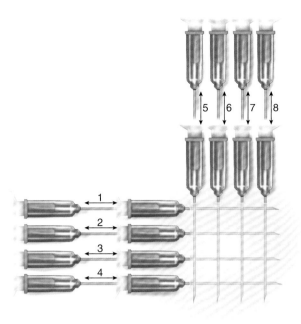

FIGURE 16 ● Cross-hatching injection technique with dermal fillers.

- **Cross-hatching.** Multiple insertion points are used to form a grid pattern of linear threads placing dermal filler product in a square area. Insert the needle at the desired tissue depth, advance the needle to the hub, and inject filler in a linear thread as the needle is fully withdrawn. Reinsert the needle in an adjacent area and place another linear thread parallel to the first thread. Repeat at 90 degrees to the first filler threads until desired correction is achieved (Fig. 16).
- **Layering.** Dermal filler product with more structural support (e.g., CaHA) is injected first in the mid- to deep dermis to treat areas of deep volume loss, using one of the above techniques. A thinner, more malleable dermal filler product (e.g., HA) is then injected in the superficial to mid-dermis overlying the first product to treat superficial wrinkles, using one of the above techniques (see Layering Dermal Fillers chapter).
- **Depot.** A single insertion point is used to place a collection of product in tissue. This technique is often used at the supraperiosteal level and is described here. A 28-gauge, ¾-inch needle is inserted through the skin and muscle and advanced until a gentle tap is felt against bone. The needle is then withdrawn 1 mm and a bolus of dermal filler product is administered just above the bone (Fig. 17). The volume injected is determined by the dermal filler product used and by the depth of the needle in the tissue. Deeper injection sites receive greater volumes. Below are listed typical depot injection volumes using a CaHA filler, Radiesse.

  If the 28-gauge, ¾-inch needle is inserted to:
- full depth, inject 0.2–0.3 mL of Radiesse
- half depth or less, inject 0.1 mL of Radiesse

Release the plunger pressure just before pulling the needle out of the skin to avoid tracking dermal filler product in the epidermis.

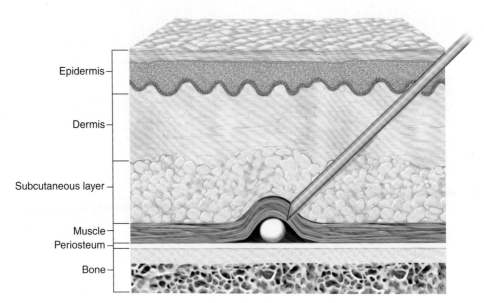

**FIGURE 17** ● Depot injection technique with dermal fillers.

## Aftercare

Direct the patient to apply a wrapped ice pack to treatment areas for 10–15 minutes every 1–2 hours and continue for 1–3 days, or until swelling and bruising resolve. Advise patients to avoid activities that can cause facial flushing such as heat application, alcohol consumption, exercising, and tanning until swelling resolves. Acetaminophen may be used if needed for discomfort. Elevating the head overnight postprocedure can reduce swelling. Advise patients against self-massaging dermal filler.

## Results and Follow-up

Dermal filler procedures yield immediate results. Providers can show patients these immediate improvements in the mirror after half the face is treated or at the end of the treatment. The duration of results is dependent upon several factors including the type of product and volume used, the patient's metabolism, degree of motion in the treatment area due to facial expressivity. In addition, dermal filler injected too deeply in the subcutaneous layer may have a shorter than intended duration, and filler injected too superficially may last longer than intended. HA dermal filler effects typically last 4–12 months, depending on the specific HA product used, and CaHA dermal filler effects typically last 12–18 months. Subsequent injection in the treatment area to maintain results is recommended when the volume of dermal filler product visibly diminishes but is still palpable, before the area returns to its pretreatment appearance. Timely subsequent treatments usually require less dermal filler product, as residual volume from the previous treatment is still present.

## Learning the Techniques

- Dermal filler injection techniques such as linear threading, fanning, cross-hatching, and depot can be practiced initially using clear silicon packs or synthetic skin models, which may be obtained from dermal filler manufacturers. However, practicing dermal filler injection on patients is necessary to acquire skill with placing product at the correct level and to gain a feel for product flow characteristics in natural tissue.

- Starting with hyaluronic acid dermal filler products that have the least resistant flow characteristics is advisable (e.g., Prevelle Silk or Juvederm Ultra XC). Hyaluronic acid treatments are also potentially correctable with the use of hyaluronidase.
- Treatment of the nasolabial folds is an ideal area to start with as the tissue is easily compressible if necessary. Beginning treatments with staff and family provides an opportunity to obtain feedback and observe the full course of a dermal filler treatment.
- Use of conservative dermal filler volumes is recommended initially as additional volume may be injected at a follow-up procedure 4 weeks after treatment if further correction is necessary.
- Once proficiency is acquired with basic dermal filler treatments, providers may choose to perform advanced filler treatments, most of which use longer lasting, more structural products (e.g., Radiesse or Perlane). When getting started with Radiesse, the technique outlined in the Layering Dermal Fillers chapter for treatment of nasolabial folds can be used without superficial layering of a second product.

## Follow-ups and Management

Patients are assessed 4 weeks after treatment to evaluate for reduction of lines and wrinkles and correction of contours. Common issues experienced by patients during this time include:

- Erythema
- Swelling
- Tenderness
- Bruising

   **Erythema, swelling, tenderness,** and **bruising** are expected after dermal filler procedures. Application of a soft, wrapped ice pack to the treatment area can minimize swelling and bruising and may be applied immediately after treatment and repeated as outlined in the Aftercare section above. Swelling typically resolves in 1–3 days and bruising may last 7–10 days, depending on the size of the bruise. Bruising can be concealed with makeup (Fig. 18). Specific colors can counter bruises at different stages: peach minimizes blue and lilac minimizes yellow discoloration. Patients who are known to have significant swelling with dermal filler injections may benefit from pretreatment with an oral over-the-counter antihistamine (e.g., cetirizine 10 mg, one tablet daily) the day of treatment, which can be continued until swelling resolves. Over-the-counter remedies that may help support healing and reduce bruising and swelling are *Arnica montana*, vitamin K, bromelain, copper, vitamin A, vitamin C, and zinc.

## Storage and Usage of Partially Used Dermal Filler Syringes

It is not uncommon to have residual dermal filler product in a syringe after treatment, especially if small volumes are required for treatment. Most package inserts that accompany dermal fillers advise against saving and, at a later date, treating with partially used syringes. One of the main concerns is possible bacterial contamination and increased risk of patient infection. A recent retrospective study evaluated infectious complications

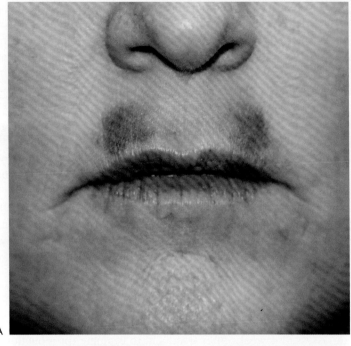

A

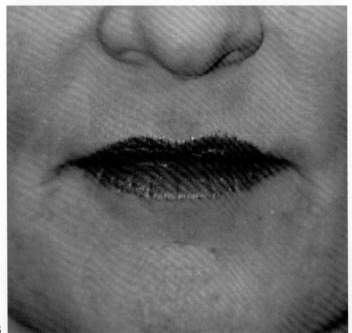

B

*FIGURE 18* ● Bruise before (**A**) and after (**B**) makeup application.

associated with the use of residual HA dermal filler product (Juvederm and Restylane) that had been refrigerated at 4°C (39°F) for approximately 6 months and found no associated infections.

## New Products and Current Developments

Beletero® is a new HA dermal filler product distributed by Merz currently used in Europe, which is undergoing trials in the United Sates. It has an expected duration of 6–9 months.

## Financial Considerations

| CPT Codes | |
| --- | --- |
| 11950 | Subcutaneous injection of filling material ≤1mL |
| 11951 | Subcutaneous injection of filling material 1.1–5.0 mL |
| 11952 | Subcutaneous injection of filling material 5.1–10 mL |

Cosmetic dermal filler treatments are typically not covered by insurance. Dermal filler fees are based on the type of filler used, size and number of syringes, the injector's skill, and vary according to community pricing in different geographic regions. Prices range from $500 to $650 per syringe of 0.8-mL HA dermal filler and from $650 to $1200 per syringe of 1.5-mL CaHA dermal filler.

## Combining Aesthetic Treatments

Facial aging is a multifaceted process involving not only the formation of facial lines and wrinkles but also contour changes, skin laxity, pigmented and vascular lesions, undesired hair growth, as well as benign and malignant degenerative changes. Achieving optimal rejuvenation results often requires a combination of minimally invasive aesthetic treatment to address these different aspects of aging. Dermal fillers can be easily combined with other procedures such as botulinum toxin to treat dynamic lines; lasers and intense pulsed light for hair reduction, skin resurfacing and treatment of benign pigmented and vascular lesion; exfoliation procedures such as microdermabrasion and chemical peels; and topical skin care products. The combination of dermal fillers and botulinum toxin may also offer advantages of longer filler duration and improve filler smoothness in highly mobile areas such as the lips and frown.

# Anesthesia

Rebecca Small, M.D.

Providing adequate anesthesia is an essential part of performing dermal filler procedures and successfully incorporating them into practice. In addition to offering the patient a better procedural experience, minimizing discomfort allows for greater dermal filler injection precision and optimal results.

Anesthesia for dermal filler treatments ideally achieves the desired anesthetic effect with minimal distortion of the treatment area, to preserve baseline tissue architecture. The main anesthesia methods for use with the dermal filler procedures in this book are reviewed below.

## Anesthesia Methods for Dermal Filler Treatments

- Injectable
  - Local infiltration
  - Ring blocks
- Topical
- Ice and other coolants

The anesthetic method chosen is dependent on the sensitivity of the treatment area, patient tolerance for pain, and the need to preserve baseline anatomy. Patients who have never had injectable cosmetic treatments typically have higher anxiety levels, lower pain tolerance, and often require injectable anesthetics to achieve adequate anesthesia. Patients with high pain thresholds and those with less anxiety around injectable procedures can often be made comfortable with topical anesthetics or topical coolants, particularly when lidocaine-based dermal fillers are used which have less procedural discomfort. Sensitive areas, such as the lips, almost always require injectable anesthesia regardless of the patient's baseline pain threshold. Each chapter recommends one method of anesthesia for use with a given procedure. However, other methods reviewed in this section may be used alternatively or adjunctively, on the basis of the patient's pain tolerance and provider preference.

Before administering anesthesia several preparatory steps are taken, which are outlined in the Preprocedure Checklist that follows.

## Preprocedure Checklist

- Confirm that the patient has no history of allergies to anesthetics or adverse responses with injectable procedures.
- Confirm that the patient has had recent food intake. If none in the last 3–4 hours offer the patient a snack, such as a granola bar or juice, to reduce the risk of hypoglycemia.
- Address anxiety symptoms and defer the procedure if the patient is excessively apprehensive.
- Obtain informed consent (for details, see Aesthetic Consultation and Preprocedure Checklist in the Introduction and Foundation Concepts section).

# Injectable Anesthetics

Lidocaine is the most commonly used injectable anesthetic for dermal filler treatments. It has a rapid onset of effect for pain inhibition within a few minutes of injection. Pressure, touch, and temperature sensations are also inhibited but the onset of these effects is slower than for pain reduction. Injectable anesthesia methods for dermal filler procedures described in this book include local infiltration and ring blocks, and are described in detail below.

## Maximum Lidocaine Dose

A common injectable anesthetic used for dermal filler procedures is lidocaine 2% solution with epinephrine 1:100,000 (referred to as lidocaine-epinephrine solution); lidocaine 1% with epinephrine may be used alternatively. Lidocaine alone is a vasodilator. When mixed with the vasoconstrictor epinephrine, this combination reduces bleeding, increases the duration of anesthetic effect, and reduces the risk of systemic toxicity by localizing the lidocaine to the injection area. Lidocaine injection volumes necessary for dermal filler treatments are typically small, ranging from 0.5 mL to a maximum of 6 mL, making lidocaine toxicity extremely rare. Nonetheless, it is important to know the maximal safe dosing for lidocaine, which is shown in Table 1. Above these doses, patients are at risk for neurotoxicity and cardiotoxicity.

## Allergy to Lidocaine

True allergic reactions to lidocaine are extremely rare. Most patients who report a lidocaine allergy describe a vasovagal event or epinephrine related symptoms such as tachycardia. In patients with sensitivity to epinephrine, it is advisable to use lidocaine without epinephrine and inform patients that their risk of bruising with dermal filler treatment is greater than when lidocaine-epinephrine solution is used. In rare cases, patients may report true signs of an allergic reaction such as puritis or papular outbreak with lidocaine injection. These allergic responses are usually because of the paraben preservatives found in multidose lidocaine vials. Single-use lidocaine vials do not contain parabens. A small test injection of 0.1 mL lidocaine from a multidose vial can be performed on the dorsum of the forearm to assess for an allergic response to preservatives. Some patients report an allergic reaction to Novocain (procaine hydrochloride) administered at dental visits. There is no cross-reactivity between lidocaine, which is an amide, and procaine, which is an ester.

## TABLE 1

### Maximum Dose of 2% Lidocaine (20 mg/mL)

| Lidocaine Solution | Maximum Adult Dose by Body Weight | Maximum Injection Volume for 140 lb (64 kg) Adult |
| --- | --- | --- |
| 2% lidocaine without epinephrine | 4 mg/kg | 13 mL |
| 2% lidocaine with epinephrine | 7 mg/kg | 22 mL |

## Complications with Injectable Anesthetics

Complications with injectable anesthetics include adverse responses to the procedure (which are most common), complications related to needles, and specific reactions to the compounds being injected.

- General procedure complications
  - Vasovagal episode
  - Hypoglycemia
  - Anxiety
- Injection complications
  - Bruising
  - Infection
  - Nerve injury
  - Allergic reactions (puritis and papules locally, and the remote possibility of urticaria, angioedema, and anaphylaxis)
  - Lidocaine toxicity of the central nervous system (dizziness, tongue numbness, tinnitus, diplopia, nystagmus, slurred speech, seizures, respiratory distress)
  - Lidocaine toxicity of the cardiovascular system (arrhythmias, hypotension, cardiac arrest)
  - Epinephrine adverse response (tachycardia, tremor, anxiety, local hypoperfusion)

Lidocaine toxicity is extremely unlikely with anesthesia for dermal filler treatments because of the relatively small doses that are used. Neurotoxicity and cardiotoxicity are possible with inadvertent intravascular injection, which can occur with nerve blocks as the targeted nerves are in close proximity with larger vessels.

## Techniques for Reducing Discomfort with Injectable Procedures

- Ensure injection solutions are at room temperature.
- Use small gauge needles (e.g., 30-gauge needle) and change after six or more injections to maintain a sharp needle.
- Inject slowly.
- Instruct patients to keep their eyes closed during the procedure and clearly inform them about each step of the process to prevent jumpiness.
- Distract patients by discussing something pleasant.
- Use breathing to assist with relaxation. Instruct patients to take a deep breath in and insert the needle upon exhalation.

## Equipment for Injectable Anesthetic Procedures: Local Infiltration and Ring Blocks

- General dermal filler equipment (see General Equipment in the Introduction and Foundation Concepts section)
- 1.0-mL, 3.0-mL, and 5.0-mL Luer-Lok™ tip syringes
- Lidocaine HCl 2% with epinephrine 1:100,000
- Lidocaine HCl 2% without epinephrine 1:100,000
- Sodium bicarbonate 8.4%
- 18-gauge, 1½-inch needle (to draw up)

- 30-gauge, ½-inch needle (for injection)
- Gauze 3 **3** 3 inches, nonwoven
- Alcohol pads

## Buffered Lidocaine

Lidocaine is acidic and may be buffered with sodium bicarbonate 8.4% in a 1:10 dilution to reduce the burning sensation upon injection, and is preferred by the author for increased patient comfort. Buffering of lidocaine is done immediately before injection.

To buffer a 1.0 mL total volume solution of 2% lidocaine-epinephrine 1:100,000 with sodium bicarbonate 8.4%:

- Use a 1.0-mL syringe with an 18-gauge 1½-inch needle to draw up 0.9 mL lidocaine-epinephrine solution.
- Detach the syringe from the needle hub and leave the needle in the lidocaine-epinephrine vial.
- Attach a new 18-gauge 1-½ inch needle to the same 1.0-mL syringe and draw up 0.1 mL sodium bicarbonate 8.4%, taking care not to push lidocaine into the sodium bicarbonate vial.
- Detach the syringe from the needle hub and leave the needle in the sodium bicarbonate vial.
- Mix the lidocaine-epinephrine solution by inverting the syringe and tapping, causing the air bubble to move.

### Tip

- If a white precipitate is visible in the buffered solution syringe, too much sodium bicarbonate has been added and the buffered mixture should not be used. When the pH is raised too high (pH . 7.8) by the addition of too much sodium bicarbonate, anesthetic precipitates out of solution reducing the clinical effectiveness of the anesthetic and injection of the solution may cause tissue irritation.

## Local Infiltration

Local infiltration in or adjacent to the dermal filler treatment area works well for most dermal filler treatments. However, local infiltration results in edema with tissue distortion and care should be taken to inject the smallest possible anesthetic volumes that can achieve adequate anesthesia.

### Overview of Local Lidocaine Infiltration Procedure

- Most dermal filler facial areas are adequately anesthetized with three to six injections of 0.1 mL buffered lidocaine-epinephrine solution.
- Local infiltration injections are placed subcutaneously. The skin should rise slightly upon injection but not appear dimpled.
- Local infiltration injection sites are shown for basic dermal filler treatment areas in Figure 1 and for advanced treatment areas that can be adequately anesthetized with local infiltration in Figure 2.

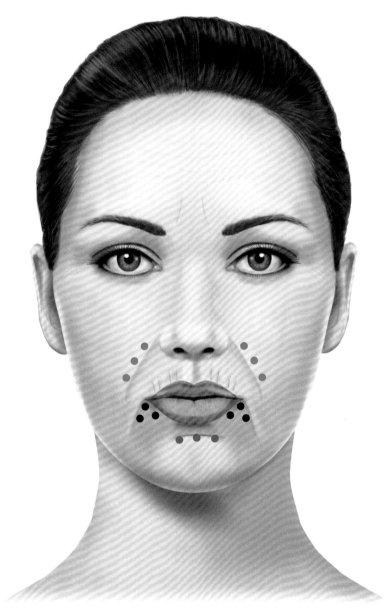

Key:

- Nasolabial fold anesthesia
- Marionette line anesthesia
- Mental crease anesthesia

All dots = 0.1 mL Lidocaine

**FIGURE 1** ● Overview of local anesthetic infiltration for basic dermal filler treatment areas.

## Performing Local Lidocaine Infiltration Procedure

- Perform the Preprocedure Checklist as outlined above.
- Using a 1.0-mL syringe and 18-gauge 1½-inch needle, draw up 1.0 mL buffered 2 % lidocaine-epinephrine solution.

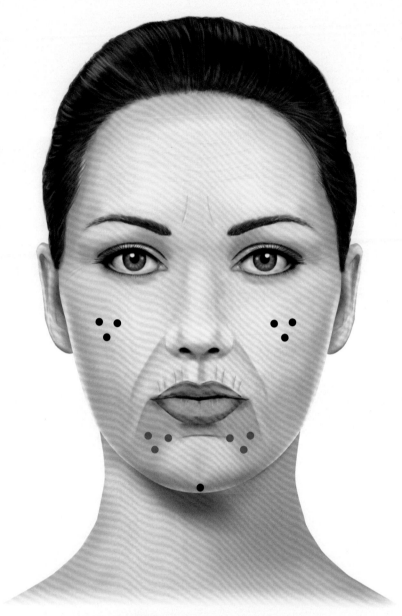

Key:
● Malar anesthesia
● Extended mental crease anesthesia
● Chin augmentation anesthesia

All dots = 0.1 mL Lidocaine

**FIGURE 2** ● Overview of local anesthetic infiltration for advanced dermal filler treatment areas.

- Change to a 30-gauge ½-inch needle.
- Prepare the skin with alcohol.
- Inject 0.1 mL buffered lidocaine-epinephrine solution subcutaneously (Fig. 3). The solution should be injected slowly to minimize discomfort.

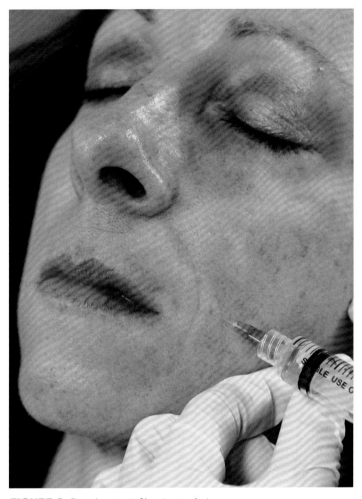

*FIGURE 3* ● Lidocaine infiltration technique.

- Proceed with subsequent injections of 0.1 mL buffered lidocaine-epinephrine solution as indicated for the specific treatment area.
- Repeat the above injections for the contralateral side of the face if required.
- Compress the injection sites away from the treatment area to minimize edema from the anesthetic.
- Allow a few minutes for the anesthetic to take effect.

## Patients with Low Pain Thresholds

Patients who have anxiety with injectable procedures, are new to your practice or have never had dermal filler treatment, often experience heightened discomfort with injections. In addition to the Techniques for Reducing Discomfort discussed above, several other techniques can aid in reducing discomfort with local infiltration:

- Pretreat the anesthetic injection sites with ice for a few minutes or another coolant such as ethyl chloride (see Ice and Other Coolants section below).

- Pretreat the anesthetic injection sites with a topical anesthetic such as benzocaine 20%: lidocaine 6%: tetracaine 4% (BLT) for 15–20 minutes prior to treatment (see Topical Anesthetics section below).

# Ring Blocks

A ring block is particularly useful with dermal filler treatment in the lip area, as it offers profound anesthesia with minimal to no distortion of the treatment area. Traditionally, nerve blocks, such as the infraorbital nerve block and mental nerve block, have been used to anesthetize lips for dermal filler treatments. These involve injection of anesthetic proximally along the nerve or at the foramen, and require larger gauge and long needles, which can be associated with greater risks. In addition, the targeted nerve may not be adequately anesthetized. Lip ring blocks are performed with short, small gauge needles and can reliably achieve upper and lower lip, as well as perioral anesthesia with minimal risks. Ring blocks are the preferred method by the author for dermal filler treatment of the lips and perioral area.

## Anatomy

- The upper and lower lips' sensory innervation is primarily from the infraorbital and mental nerves (Fig. 4; Dermal Filler Anatomy section, Fig. 4).

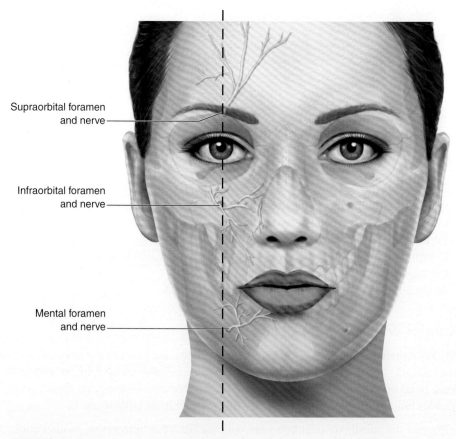

Supraorbital foramen and nerve

Infraorbital foramen and nerve

Mental foramen and nerve

*FIGURE 4* ● Nerves and foramen of the face.

- The **upper lip** is innervated by the distal portion of the inferior branch of the infraorbital nerve. The superior branches of the infraorbital nerve innervate the lower eyelid, lateral nose, and medial cheek.
- The **lower lip** is innervated by the mental nerve.
- The **corners of the lips** are innervated by the distal portion of the buccal nerve.
- The infraorbital and mental nerves lie along a vertical line that extends from the supraorbital notch to the mandible (Fig. 4). The supraorbital notch lies along the upper border of the orbit, and is palpable approximately 2.5 cm lateral to the midline of the face. The infraorbital foramen is palpable approximately 1 cm inferior to the infraorbital boney margin and the mental foramen is palpable 1 cm above the margin of the mandible.

## Overview of Lip Ring Block Procedure

- Perform Preprocedure Checklist as outlined above.
- The primary target for the upper lip ring block is the distal portion of the inferior branch of the infraorbital nerve and the primary target of lower lip ring block is the distal mental nerve. The lip ring block technique described below utilizes a short, ½-inch needle, which reaches only the distal portions of the infraorbital and mental nerves that innervate the lips.
- Lip ring block injections are intraoral and use lidocaine 2% with epinephrine 1:100,000 (buffered or unbuffered).
- **Upper lip ring block** injection sites and doses are shown in Figure 5. There are four injections for the upper lip and a total of 1.2 mL lidocaine-epinephrine solution is injected. The upper lip is more sensitive than the lower lip and anesthesia of the injection sites may also be required for patient comfort. Injection site anesthesia can be achieved using topical benzocaine before performing the ring block.

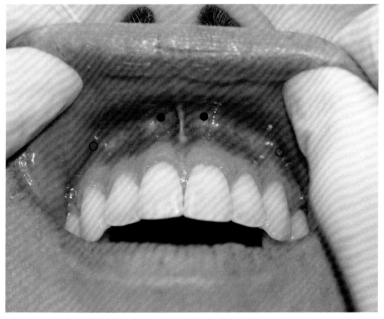

● = 0.1 mL Lidocaine    ○ = 0.5 mL Lidocaine

*FIGURE 5* ● Overview of upper lip ring block injection sites and doses.

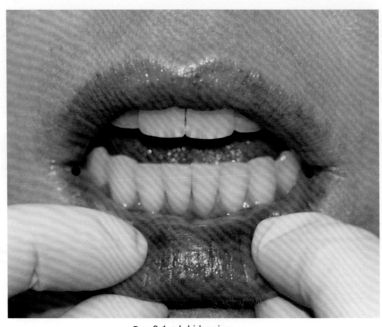

● = 0.1 mL Lidocaine

*FIGURE 6* ● Local lidocaine infiltration for anesthetizing the corners of the lips.

- **Corners of the lips** are poorly anesthetized with upper or lower lip ring blocks and require additional local lidocaine infiltration. Injection sites and doses for anesthetizing the corners of the lips are shown in Figure 6. There is one injection of 0.1 mL lidocaine-epinephrine solution at each corner.
- **Lower lip ring block** injection sites and doses are shown in Figure 7. There are four injections for the lower lip and a total of 1.2 mL lidocaine-epinephrine solution is injected.

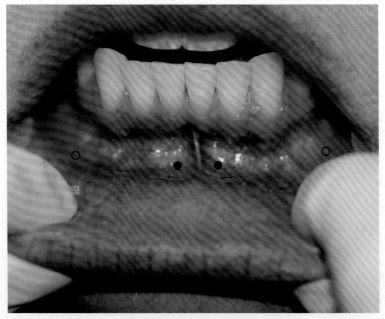

● = 0.1 mL Lidocaine      ○ = 0.5 mL Lidocaine

*FIGURE 7* ● Overview of lower lip ring block injection sites and doses.

- All lip ring block injections are placed at the gingivobuccal margin just under the submucosa, except for the injections targeting the distal branches of the infraorbital and mental nerves. These injections are placed deeper under the submucosa along the maxilla and mandible bones, respectively.

## Performing Upper Lip Ring Block Procedure

- Position the patient upright at about 60 degrees with the chin tipped upward.
- The provider is positioned on the opposite side of upper lip to be anesthetized.
- Lift the upper lip to visualize the gingivobuccal margin.
- The injection points along the gingivobuccal margin can be anesthetized with benzocaine, using either a prefilled swab (e.g., CaineTips) (Fig. 8) or a small amount of benzocaine gel 20% (e.g., Ultracare) on a cotton-tipped applicator. The swab or gel is placed along gingivobuccal margin between the frenulum and the maxillary canine tooth. Benzocaine takes effect in less than 1 minute and does not need to be removed prior to injection.
- The first upper lip injection point is at the gingivobuccal margin just lateral to the maxillary canine (third tooth from the midline). Insert a 30-gauge, ½-inch needle under the mucosa and direct the needle superiorly toward the pupil, staying parallel to the maxilla. Advance the needle almost the full length and inject 0.5 mL lidocaine (Fig. 9). The anesthetic should flow easily. If the needle is angled too superficially, lidocaine may be placed in the dermis which can be felt as resistance during injection. After removing the needle, compress the deep palpable wheal of lidocaine superiorly toward the infraorbital foramen.
- The second upper lip injection point is just lateral to the upper lip frenulum. Insert the needle tip just under the mucosa and inject 0.1 mL lidocaine (Fig. 10). After the needle is removed, compress the injection site to distribute the lidocaine.

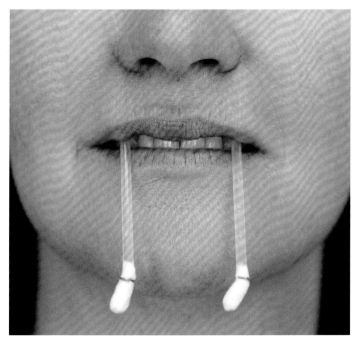

*FIGURE 8* ● Benzocaine swabs.

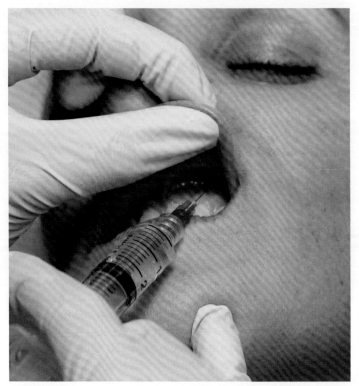

*FIGURE 9* ● First lidocaine injection for upper lip ring block.

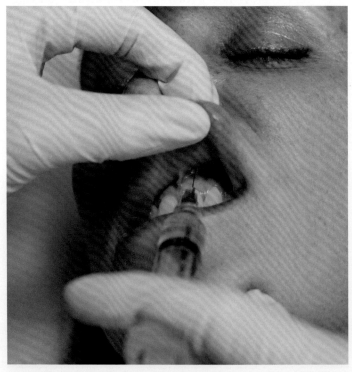

*FIGURE 10* ● Second lidocaine injection for upper lip ring block.

- Perform injections for the corners of lips as described below.
- Reposition to the opposite side and repeat earlier injections to anesthetize the contralateral upper lip.
- Anesthetic effect typically takes 5–10 minutes.
- Test sensation of the upper lip before initiating dermal filler treatment. If adequate anesthesia is not achieved, repeat the procedure injecting an additional 0.5 mL lidocaine at the maxillary canine injection site and wait an additional 10 minutes.

## Performing Local Infiltration Injections for Corners of Lips

- The provider is positioned on the opposite side of the corner to be injected.
- Insert the needle tip just under the mucosa and inject 0.1 mL lidocaine (Fig. 11).
- After the needle is removed, compress the injection site to distribute the lidocaine.
- Reposition to the opposite side and repeat the above injection.

## Performing Lower Lip Ring Block Procedure

- Position patient upright at about 60 degrees with chin tipped downward.
- The provider is positioned on the opposite side of the lower lip to be anesthetized.
- Lift the lower lip to visualize the gingivobuccal margin.
- The first lower lip injection point is at the gingivobuccal margin just lateral to the first mandibular bicuspid (also called the first premolar, which is the fourth tooth from the midline). Insert a 30-gauge, ½-inch needle under the mucosa and direct the needle inferiorly toward the mental foramen, staying parallel to the mandible. Advance the needle half way and inject 0.5 mL lidocaine (Fig. 12). The anesthetic

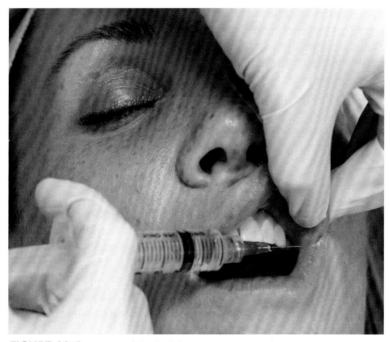

**FIGURE 11** ● Corner of the lip lidocaine injection technique.

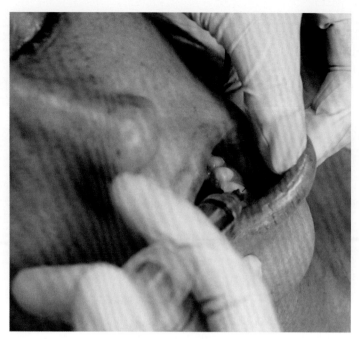

FIGURE 12 ● Lower lip ring block injection technique.

should flow easily unless the needle is angled too superficially into the dermis. After removing the needle, compress the deep palpable wheal of lidocaine inferiorly toward the mental foramen.

- The second lower lip injection point is just lateral to the lower lip frenulum. Insert the needle tip just under the mucosa and inject 0.1 mL lidocaine. After the needle is removed, compress the injection site to distribute the lidocaine.
- If the upper lip ring block procedure was not performed, then proceed with injections for the corners of the lips as described in the previous section.
- Reposition to the opposite side and repeat the earlier injections to anesthetize the contralateral lower lip.
- Anesthetic effect typically takes 5–10 minutes.
- Test sensation of the lower lip before initiating dermal filler treatment. If adequate anesthesia is not achieved, repeat the procedure injecting an additional 0.5 mL lidocaine at the first mandibular bicuspid injection site and wait an additional 10 minutes.

## Topical Anesthetics

Topical anesthetics are often used with dermal filler procedures due to their ease of application. With the incorporation of lidocaine into dermal filler products, discomfort with dermal filler treatment has been reduced. Some patients, particularly those with high pain thresholds, can tolerate treatment with a dermal filler product plus lidocaine using only a topical anesthetic or topical coolant for anesthesia.

Topical anesthetics have the same mechanism of action as injectable anesthetics with blocking sensory nerves through neuronal impulse inhibition, and they reduce discomfort associated with needle insertion. Table 2 shows commonly used topical anesthetic products. BLT is one of the most potent and fast acting topical anesthetics

## TABLE 2

**Commonly Used Topical Anesthetic Products for Dermal Filler Procedures**

- L-M-X (lidocaine 4%–5%)[a]
- EMLA (lidocaine 2.5%:prilocaine 2.5%)[b]
- BLT (benzocaine 20%:lidocaine 6%:tetracaine 4%)[c]

[a]Over-the-counter product
[b]Prescription
[c]Compounded by a pharmacy
See Appendix 5 for suppliers

and is preferred for use by the author. It is applied in-office, with a maximum dose of 0.5 g and is typically applied for 15 minutes. Some providers enhance topical anesthetic effects by occluding the product under plastic wrap once applied to the skin, however, due to its potency, occlusion under plastic wrap is not necessary with BLT. Some pharmacies formulate BLT with the vasoconstrictor phenylephrine, which may reduce the risk of systemic toxicity through localizing the BLT to the application area, similar to epinephrine's effect with lidocaine.

## Dosing

The local effect of a topical anesthetic is related to the concentration of ingredients, surface area, duration of application, and penetration into the skin.

The dosing of BLT is limited by the concentration of tetracaine, as this agent has the greatest toxicity risk. Tetracaine 4% corresponds to 40 mg/g. An application of 0.5 g BLT contains 20 mg tetracaine, which is the maximal recommended dose (Table 3). BLT products formulated with phenylephrine may have different maximal doses and it is advisable to ascertain the maximal dose of the specific BLT product used from the compounding pharmacy.

## Complications with Topical Anesthetics

The application surface area is small with dermal filler treatments, and consequently, there are few reported complications with topical anesthetics applied to the face. Cases

## TABLE 3

**Maximum Dose of Topical Anesthetics**

| Topical Anesthetic | Maximum Adult Dose | Time to Peak | Duration of Effect |
|---|---|---|---|
| Lidocaine | 500 mg/dose | 2–5 min | 30 min |
| Lidocaine with prilocaine | 60 mg/dose | 60–120 min | 90 min |
| Tetracaine | 20 mg/dose | 3–8 min | 45 min |

of toxicity with topical anesthetics have been reported with application to large surface areas, such as full lower extremities prior to laser hair reduction treatments, and with fractional ablative laser treatments where skin is not intact. Possible topical anesthetic complications are listed as follows:

- Allergic reactions (puritis and papules locally, and the remote possibility of urticaria, angioedema, and anaphylaxis).
- Lidocaine toxicity of the central nervous system (dizziness, tongue numbness, tinnitus, diplopia, nystagmus, slurred speech, seizures, respiratory distress).
- Lidocaine toxicity of the cardiovascular system (arrhythmias, hypotension, cardiac arrest).
- Tetracaine toxicity of the central nervous system (restlessness, agitation, seizure activity).
- Lidocaine, tetracaine, or prilocaine can cause methemoglobinemia (cyanosis, acidosis).

### Equipment for Topical Anesthetics

- Topical anesthetic
- Alcohol pads
- Plastic wrap (for occlusion of topical anesthetic)

### Performing Topical Anesthetic Procedure

- Perform Preprocedure Checklist as outlined above.
- Prepare the skin in the treatment area using alcohol to degrease the skin and enhance anesthetic penetration.
- Apply the topical anesthetic to the skin in the treatment area using a gloved finger or cotton-tipped applicator and rub gently to enhance penetration. Figure 13 shows a patient with BLT on half the face (for demonstration purposes).
- If not using BLT, occlude topical anesthetic under plastic wrap to enhance penetration.
- Remove all topical anesthetic with alcohol after 15 to 30 minutes, depending on the topical anesthetic used.

## Ice and Other Coolants

Ice and other topical coolant modalities are anesthetic options that may be used as alternatives to or adjunctively with other anesthesia methods listed above. These include:

- Ice packs
- Vapocoolant (e.g., ethyl chloride spray)
- Contact cooling device (e.g., ArTek® Spot)

### Equipment for Ice and Topical Coolants

- Ice or coolant
- Alcohol
- Power source for contact cooling devices

### Performing Ice and Topical Coolant Procedures

- **Ice** may be applied to the skin immediately before injection for approximately 1–2 minutes, until the skin is erythematous but not blanched (Fig. 14). Prepare the skin in the treatment area using alcohol.

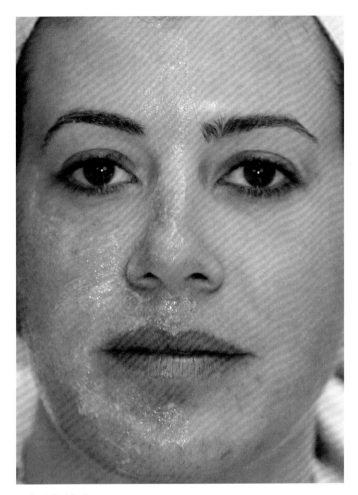

*FIGURE 13* ● Topical anesthetic.

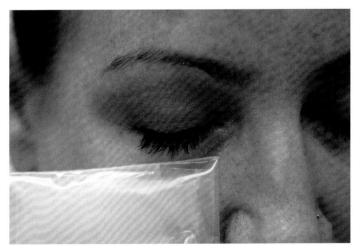

*FIGURE 14* ● Ice.

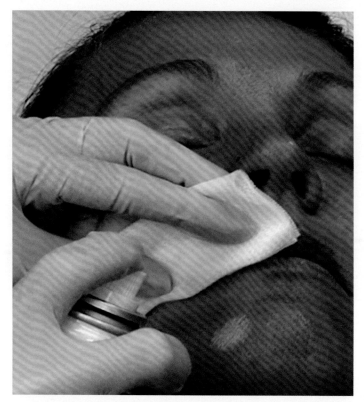

FIGURE 15 ● Vapocoolant (ethyl chloride spray).

- **Vapocoolant,** such as ethyl chloride (e.g., Pain Ease), may be sprayed immediately before treatment by holding the can upright 3–4 inches from the injection site and spraying for about 5 seconds until the skin just turns white (Fig. 15). Prepare the skin with alcohol.
- **Contact cooling devices** (e.g., ArTek Spot) can be used in place of ice or a vapocoolant. Anesthesia is achieved by applying contact cooling immediately before treatment for approximately 1–2 minutes or until the skin is erythematous. Prepare the skin in the treatment area using alcohol.

## Tip

- The goal temperature for contact cooling is approximately 5°C. Over cooling with prolonged blanching of the skin can result in epidermal injury.

# Complications

### Rebecca Small, M.D.

Transient postinjection erythema, swelling, tenderness, and bruising are expected with dermal filler treatments, and are considered part of routine follow-up rather than complications. These issues and suggestions for management are reviewed in Follow-ups and Management of the Introduction and Foundation Concepts section.

Each dermal filler product has specific side effects and complications associated with their use. The following section focuses on complications seen with hyaluronic acid (HA) and calcium hydroxylapatite (CaHA) which, relative to other dermal filler products, have comparatively good safety profiles. Severe product-related complications such as granulomatous reactions are extremely rare with temporary dermal fillers such as these, and are more commonly reported with permanent dermal fillers such as silicone, polymethylmethacrylate (ArteFill®), and certain semipermanent fillers such as poly-L-lactic acid (Sculptra®).

## Complications

- Extensive bruising or rarely, hematoma
- Visible or palpable filler bumpiness
- Asymmetry, overcorrection, or undercorrection
- Unpredictable persistence of filler, either shorter or longer than anticipated
- Tyndall effect (bluish discoloration)
- Migration or extrusion of filler
- Prolonged or severe swelling
- Prolonged erythema
- Hyperpigmentation and rare possibility of hypopigmentation
- Infection (e.g., reactivation of herpes simplex or herpes zoster, bacterial infection)
- Erythematous, tender bumps, and nodules
- Granulomas
- Keratoacanthomas
- Tissue ischemia and skin necrosis
- Blindness
- Allergic hypersensitivity reactions (e.g., urticaria, angioedema, and a remote possibility of anaphylaxis)
- Scarring

**Extensive bruising** (Fig. 1) can occur when dermal filler is injected in a large region, when extensive fanning or cross-hatching is performed, or if a large blood vessel is nicked. It occurs most often in patients taking anti-inflammatory medications such as acetylsalicylic acid (Aspirin). Extravasated blood can migrate to dependent areas, which is seen several days after the initial bruise. The use of small gauge needles with gentle injection technique, and avoidance of anti-inflammatory medications and other supplements with anticoagulant effects prior to procedures, can help reduce bruising. Bruises may be camouflaged with makeup. See Follow-ups and Management in the Introduction and Foundation Concepts section for more information about bruising and management.

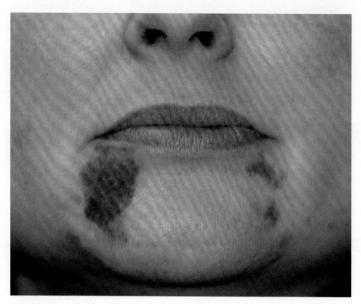

*FIGURE 1* ● Extensive bruising, 2 days after dermal filler treatment (Radiesse®, a semipermanent calcium hydroxylapatite product).

**Filler bumpiness** evident at the time of, or shortly after treatment, is a complication related to injection technique and volumes. It is usually caused by placement of filler too superficially or unevenly. Dermal fillers with more structural support, such as CaHA, are more likely to cause bumpiness than thinner, more malleable fillers such as HAs. **Bumpiness** and areas of **overcorrection** resolve as filler volume diminishes. If patients are distressed, these filler collections can often be corrected with vigorous compression by the provider (see General Injection Principles in the Introduction and Foundation Concepts section). Compression may result in bruising, and local anesthesia may be required at the time of filler compression for patient comfort. Lancing of large filler collections with a scalpel and expressing the product has also been reported. Increasingly, providers are using hyaluronidase (5–20 units initially) for correction of HA collections as well as treatment of other HA complications such as vascular compromise (see Hyaluronidase section later).

**Asymmetry** and **undercorrection** result from unbalanced injection volumes or injecting too little dermal filler. These complications can occur with patients who exhibit rapid swelling during dermal filler treatment; however, they are more often related to injectors' skill and experience. Additional filler may be necessary for correction and it is important to discuss this possibility with patients prior to initial dermal filler treatment due to the cost associated with this unanticipated procedure.

**Filler persistence can be unpredictable**, either shorter or longer than anticipated, and can vary from the dermal filler product's FDA approved duration. Product persistence in tissue tends to decrease with small injection volumes, highly mobile treatment areas, and in patients with a high metabolism.

**Tyndall effect**, seen as a bluish discoloration of the skin, may occur with superficial placement of HA in thin-skinned areas, such as the tear trough area. Areas with the Tyndall effect can be managed with compression, hyaluronidase injection, or treatment with a Q-switched 1064-nm laser.

**Migration** of dermal filler may occur with aggressive post-procedure massaging. It is therefore, advisable to instruct patients to avoid palpating the treatment area. **Extrusion** could possibly occur shortly after treatment from a needle insertion site.

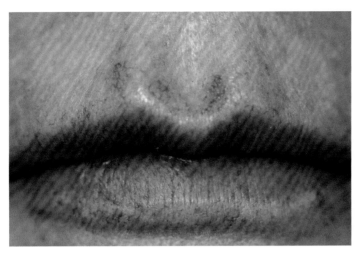

*FIGURE 2* ● Prolonged erythema, several years after dermal filler treatment (Restylane®, a long acting product).

**Prolonged swelling** may be seen for up to 4 weeks after treatment in some patients, without associated tenderness, pain, or bumps. The swelling is typically small but clinically evident. Prolonged swelling is more common if extensive bruising has occurred with treatment. Ice and oral antihistamines (e.g., cetirizine 10 mg, one tablet daily) may be used until swelling resolves (see Aftercare in the Introduction and Foundation Concepts section). In rare cases of **severe swelling** and **allergic hypersensitivity** reactions, such as **urticaria** and **angioedema**, intramuscular steroids (dexamethasone 8 mg) followed by oral steroids (prednisone 60 mg per day tapered over 1–2 weeks) may be necessary.

**Prolonged erythema** without other associated signs of tenderness, pain, bumps, or swelling, can be seen as hypervascularity overlying the dermal filler treatment area (Figs. 2 and 3). Lasers or intense pulsed light devices specific for reduction of vascularities

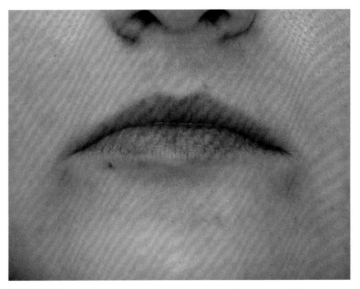

*FIGURE 3* ● Prolonged erythema, 3 months after dermal filler treatment (Evolence™, a semipermanent collagen filler).

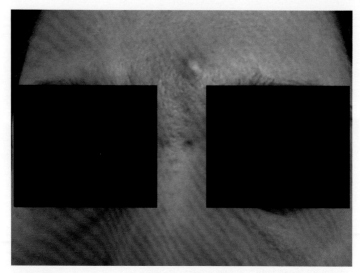

*FIGURE 4* ● Infectious nodule, 2 weeks after dermal filler treatment (Aquamid®, a permanent polyacrylamide filler) (Courtesy of L. H. Christensen, M.D.).

can be effective in reducing erythema. Prolonged erythema may stimulate **postinflammatory hyperpigmentation**, which can be treated with topical lightening products such as hydroquinone.

**Infection**, such as reactivation of herpes simplex or herpes zoster can occur, and may be prevented with prophylactic antiviral medications (valacyclovir 500 mg, one tablet twice daily, taken 2 days prior to treatment and 3 days posttreatment). Anytime the skin barrier is breached bacterial or fungal infection is possible. Preparing the injection area adequately can reduce the risk of inoculating the skin with pathogens. The mouth harbors numerous bacteria and ensuring that needles are changed between lip injections and other dermal injections may also aid in reducing the risk of infection.

**Erythematous, tender bumps, and nodules** are treated as bacterial infections (Fig. 4). These can occur immediately after treatment or can be delayed up to a year or more. Management typically consists of a 6-week course of empiric antibiotics with a macrolide (e.g., clarithromycin 500 mg, one tablet twice daily) or a tetracycline (e.g., minocycline 100 mg, one tablet twice daily). Fluctuant nodules are incised, drained, and cultured before initiating antibiotics. Hyaluronidase can be injected into the nodular area if HA dermal fillers were used. There is new evidence suggesting that late-onset erythematous tender nodules may be due to biofilms, which are aggregates of microorganisms within adhesive protective coverings that can adhere to foreign bodies. Biofilms can be elusive to standard culture methods and highly resistant to antibiotics. They are presumed to resolve once the dermal filler foreign body is gone. Late-onset erythematous tender nodules are treated as above, and referral to a plastic surgeon may be necessary for excision if nodules do not resolve.

**Granulomas** are a delayed complication that typically present as tender nodules with or without fluctuance, appearing up to 2 years after treatment. They are more common with permanent fillers (Fig. 5) and certain semipermanent fillers. Some granulomas spontaneously resolve, whereas others require intralesional steroid injection or excision and consultation for management is advised if this lesion is suspected. Certain dermal filler products have higher reported incidences of granulomas and providers may want

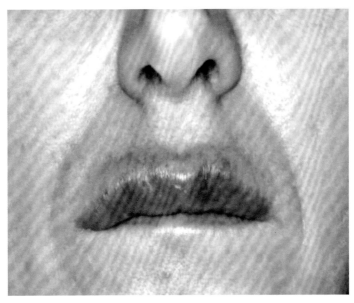

*FIGURE 5* ● Granuloma, 3 years after dermal filler treatment (Dermalive®, a permanent acrylic hydrogel filler) (Courtesy of L. H. Christensen, M.D.).

to carefully weigh the risk to benefit ratio when considering their use. Sculptra, for example, has a reported granuloma incidence as high as 13% (Fig. 6).

**Keratoacanthomas**, which are benign epithelial tumors, can arise in response to trauma and have been reported following dermal filler treatments (Fig. 7). These lesions can be refractory to treatment and it is advisable to seek consultation for management if these rare lesions arise.

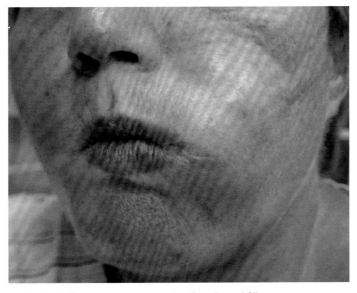

*FIGURE 6* ● Granuloma, 6 weeks after dermal filler treatment (Sculptra®, a semipermanent poly-L-lactic acid filler) (Courtesy of L. H. Christensen, M.D.).

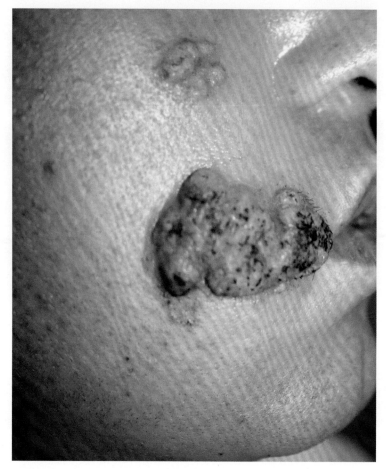

*FIGURE 7* ● Keratoacanthoma, 2 months after dermal filler treatment (collagen) (Courtesy of L. Baumann, M.D.).

**Tissue ischemia**, or reduced blood supply to tissue, is a potentially serious complication that can result in **tissue necrosis** (Fig. 8). Compromised blood flow to the treatment area can result from overfilling tissue with dermal filler or injecting intravascularly. Ischemia typically appears as a violaceous reticular pattern or white blanching of the affected area, with or without associated pain. It may be seen at the time of dermal filler injection, or delayed and has been reported up to 6 hours after treatment. High-risk areas for vascular compromise include, but are not limited to, the following:

- **Glabella.** Vascular occlusion of the supraorbital artery has been reported. In addition, this is a watershed area with limited collateral circulation and is susceptible to vascular compromise due to overfilling tissue with dermal filler. **Blindness** due to retinal artery embolization has been reported with dermal filler treatment in this area.
- **Nasal ala.** The nasal ala and tip are primarily supplied by the lateral nasal artery. Necrosis of the ala has been reported with dermal filler treatments of the nasolabial folds.
- **Superior marionette line.** This area is at risk for ischemia and necrosis due to overfilling the tissue with dermal filler rather than intravascular injection.

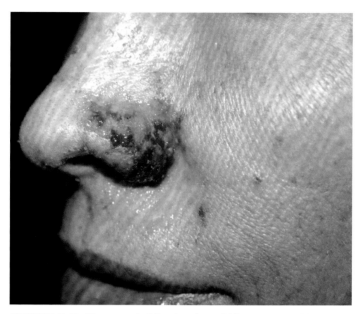

FIGURE 8 ● Alar necrosis following dermal filler treatment (Courtesy of L. Baumann, M.D.).

- **Body of the lips.** The labial arteries lie deep to the labial mucosa and are at risk for intravascular dermal filler injection.

**Ischemia** is managed urgently as it can rapidly progress to **tissue necrosis.** If ischemia occurs the following are recommended as part of management:

1. Discontinue injection immediately.
2. Attempt to revascularize the area by firmly and vigorously massaging the ischemic tissue.
3. Apply heat packs.
4. Administer 2 chewable 325 mg aspirin.
5. Apply a vasodilator, such as nitroglycerine ointment (Nitro-Bid® 2% approximately 1 inch) under occlusion with plastic wrap to the affected area. Nitroglycerine can decrease blood pressure and vital signs may need to be monitored.
6. If a HA dermal filler was used, perform a hyaluronidase skin test and if negative after 5 minutes, inject 30–50 units of hyaluronidase in the treatment area and along the course of the blood vessels in the treatment area (see Hyaluronidase section later).
7. It may be advisable to contact the local emergency room and/or a local plastic surgeon if ischemia does not rapidly resolve.

It can be helpful to have supplies assembled for treatment of ischemia in an emergency vascular occlusion kit (see Introduction and Foundation Concepts section, Fig. 16). All steps listed earlier may not be required for every ischemic event. For example, tissue ischemia in the marionette line area, which is usually due to overfilling tissue, typically resolves with discontinuing injection and massaging. However, tissue ischemia of the nasal ala, which is more likely an intravascular occlusion, may require all of the above steps to achieve revascularization. Monitoring of the ischemic area and close follow-up is advised. If an ischemic event occurs, modify the patient's dermal filler home care instructions to avoid icing the area that had vascular compromise. Necrosis may be seen a few days to weeks after an ischemic event. Nonintact skin is treated with moist wound care using an antibiotic ointment until healed.

Prevention of intravascular injection can be challenging with dermal fillers. Because of the viscous nature of dermal fillers and small gauge needles used for injection, aspiration prior to injection to ensure a vessel has not been cannulated is not feasible with dermal filler procedures. In addition, a blood "flashback" in the needle hub is also not seen if a vessel is inadvertently cannulated with dermal fillers. Gentle plunger pressure, keeping the needle moving during filler injection and using conservative dermal filler volumes for treatment may reduce the risk of ischemia because of intravascular injection or overfilling of tissues.

**Scarring** is rare with dermal filler treatments, but may occur with any injection, particularly if the treatment is complicated by infection. Patients with a history of overhealing responses such as hypertrophic and keloidal scarring are at increased risk. Injections performed with very large gauge needles, such as those used with autologous fat dermal filler injections, can be associated with scarring (Fig. 9).

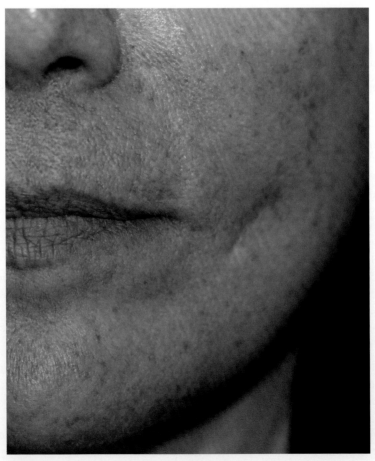

*FIGURE 9* ● Scar, 1 year after dermal filler treatment (autologous fat).

# Hyaluronidase

Hyaluronidase is an enzyme that breaks down HA and it is an emerging therapy used for correction of HA dermal filler complications such as filler bumpiness and vascular compromise. Hyaluronidase is not currently FDA approved for these indications.

## Hyaluronidase Off-label Indications

- Bumpiness and overcorrection due to HA injection
- Tyndall effect due to HA injection
- Tissue ischemia due to HA injection
- Nodules and granulomatous reactions due to HA injection

## Hyaluronidase Contraindications

- Allergy to bee stings (bee venom has hyaluronidase)
- Known hypersensitivity to hyaluronidase or its components
- Current use of furosemide, epinephrine, benzodiazepines, heparin or phenytoin
- Pregnancy

## Hyaluronidase Products

Hyaluronidase is available as a powder or solution. Powdered hyaluronidase is reconstituted with sterile normal saline and is used within 12 hours of reconstitution. Hyaluronidase solutions must be refrigerated. Commercially available hyaluronidase is either bovine (cow) or ovine (sheep) derived (see Table 1). Hylenex, a human recombinant hyaluronidase, has been recalled by the manufacturer but may be available in the future. Product dosing is equivalent for the different hyaluronidases listed below.

## Hyaluronidase Complications

Use of hyaluronidase for management of HA complications has not been widely studied and there are sparse data on complication rates. Most adverse reactions are local. Rarely, allergic reactions such as urticaria, angioedema, and anaphylaxis have been reported.

## TABLE 1

**Hyaluronidase Products**

| Agent | Source | Other Ingredients | Concentration |
| --- | --- | --- | --- |
| Amphadase® | Bovine | Thimerosal (preservative) | 150 units/mL |
| Vitrase® | Ovine | Albumin | 200 units/mL |

### Hyaluronidase Skin Testing

Skin testing is recommended for all hyaluronidase products to ensure there is no allergic reaction to the product or its components. If a positive reaction is observed, hyaluronidase is contraindicated.

1. Draw up 3 units of hyaluronidase (0.02 mL of 150 unit/mL solution).
2. Inject subdermally on the dorsum of the forearm.
3. Evaluate in 5 minutes. A positive reaction includes any of the following: palpable wheal, induration, local puritis, or systemic allergic signs (urticaria, angioedema, and anaphylaxis).

### Hyaluronidase Dosing

- Hyaluronic acid dermal filler bumpiness, overcorrection, Tyndall effect nodules, or granulomas: 5–20 units initially, injected intradermally in the HA collection.
- Vascular occlusion: 30–50 units initially, injected intradermally and subcutaneously along the course of the artery.

There is a concern that high hyaluronidase doses may degrade native dermal HA resulting in soft tissue depressions. However, this has not yet been rigorously studied. Some providers report use of doses as high as 375 units without adverse changes in facial volume.

### Timing of Hyaluronidase Effects

Data are sparse regarding hyaluronidase pharmacokinetics, but evidence suggests that the time for onset of effects may be dose dependent. With conservative hyaluronidase doses of 5–20 units used to treat HA collections, smoothing effects may be fully evident 1–2 weeks after injection. With high hyaluronidase doses of 150–200 units, effects may be evident within hours of injection.

## Conclusion

All dermal filler treatments have associated risks of complications. These reactions vary from erythema and edema to more serious complications of necrosis and even blindness. Whereas severe adverse reactions are rare, appraising patients of all possible complications is essential prior to dermal filler treatment.

# Treatment Areas

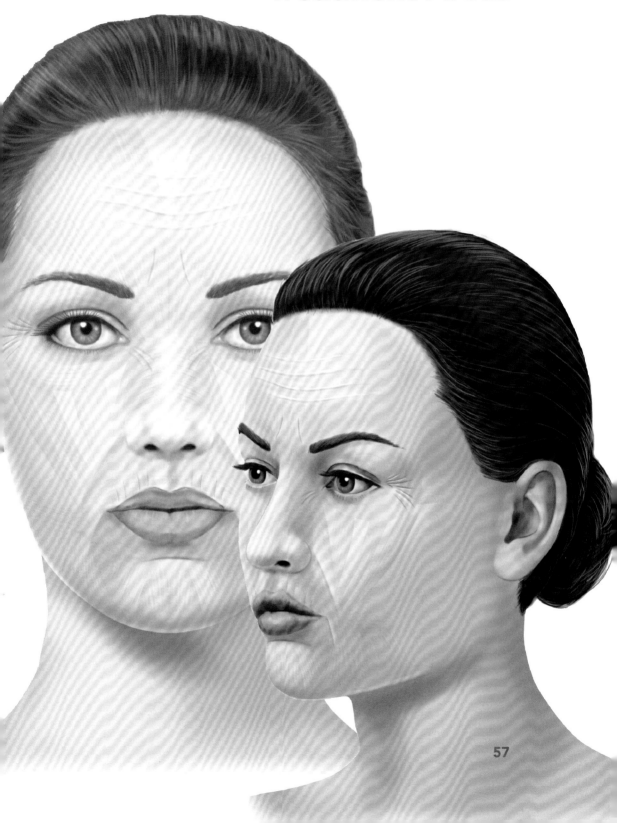

# Chapter 1

# Nasolabial Folds

Rebecca Small, M.D.

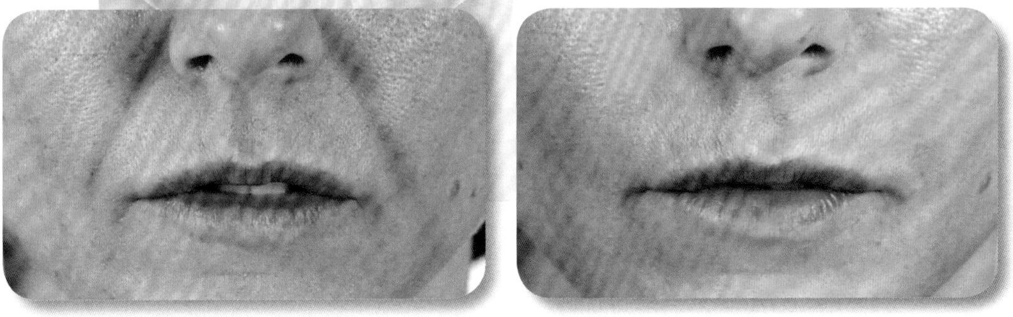

**FIGURE 1** ● Nasolabial folds before **(A)** and 2 weeks after **(B)** dermal filler treatment, using hyaluronic acid.

Nasolabial folds are natural facial contours that can become more prominent with age, projecting a fatigued or drawn appearance. Reduction of the nasolabial folds is one of the most commonly performed dermal filler treatments.

## Indications

• Nasolabial folds

## Anatomy

**Wrinkles, folds, and contours.** Nasolabial folds, or melolabial folds, course diagonally in the midface from the nasal ala toward the corner of the lip (see Dermal Filler Anatomy section, Figs. 1 and 2). Many factors contribute to nasolabial fold formation including soft tissue volume loss and dermal atrophy, reduced skin elasticity, descent of malar fat pads, and hyperdynamic midface musculature. The lateral nasal artery is the main vascular supply for the nasal tip and ala. It is in close proximity to the nasolabial fold, 2–3 mm superior to the alar groove (see Dermal Filler Anatomy section, Figs. 3 and 5).

## Patient Assessment

- Patients with mild, moderate, and severe static nasolabial folds are candidates for dermal filler treatments.
- Patients presenting with excess laxity and hanging skin folds usually require surgical intervention for significant improvement.

## Contraindications

- See Contraindications in the Introduction and Foundation Concepts section.

## Treatment Goals

- Reduction of nasolabial folds without full effacement.

## Recommended Dermal Filler Product

- Basic hyaluronic acid (HA) dermal filler products that have lidocaine (HA-lidocaine) are recommended for treatment of nasolabial folds, such as Juvederm® Ultra XC, Juvederm® Ultra Plus XC or Restylane-L® (see Basic and Advanced Procedures in the Introduction and Foundation Concepts section).
- This chapter describes treatment of nasolabial folds with Juvederm Ultra Plus XC (HA-lidocaine).

## Dermal Filler Treatment Volumes

- The estimated HA dermal filler volume necessary for treatment is based on the patient's observed facial anatomy and volume loss in the treatment area. Typical starting volumes are listed as follows:
  - Mild nasolabial folds typically require a total volume of 0.8-mL HA-lidocaine.
  - Moderate nasolabial folds typically require a total volume of 1.6-mL HA-lidocaine.
  - Severe nasolabial folds typically require a total volume of 2.4-mL HA-lidocaine.

## Equipment for Anesthesia

- Local infiltration injection supplies (see Equipment for Injectable Anesthetics in the Anesthesia section)
- Lidocaine HCl 2% with epinephrine 1:100,000 buffered (referred to as buffered 2% lidocaine-epinephrine solution)
- 30-gauge, ½-inch needle

## Equipment for Dermal Filler Procedure

- General dermal filler injection supplies (see Equipment in the Introduction and Foundation Concepts section)
- 30-gauge, ½-inch needle

## Anesthesia Overview

- **Local lidocaine infiltration.** Buffered 2% lidocaine-epinephrine solution can be used to achieve anesthesia for nasolabial folds.
- Both folds are anesthetized using six injections of 0.1 mL for a total volume of 0.6 mL (Fig. 2).

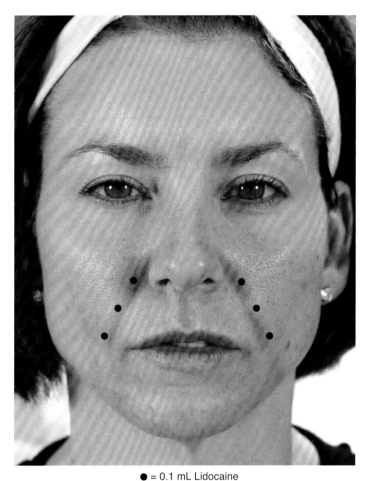

● = 0.1 mL Lidocaine

*FIGURE 2* ● Anesthesia for nasolabial fold dermal filler treatment.

See Injectable Anesthetics in the Anesthesia section for additional information on local infiltration methods. Sensitivity increases with proximity to the nose and anesthetic injections are started at the inferior portion of the fold.

- **Topical anesthetic.** Benzocaine:lidocaine:tetracaine (BLT) may be used as an alternative for patients with high pain thresholds (see Topical Anesthetics in the Anesthesia section).

## Dermal Filler Procedure Overview

- **Overview.** An overview of injection points and injection technique for treatment of nasolabial folds, using a HA dermal filler is shown in Figure 3.
- **Number of injections.** There are two linear thread injections and one fanning injection per side (see Techniques for Dermal Filler Injection in the Introduction and Foundation Concepts section). All injections are placed medial to the nasolabial folds. Injections start at the inferior most portion of the nasolabial fold and proceed superiorly toward the nose.
- **Injection depth.** Dermal filler is injected in the mid- to deep dermis for treatment of nasolabial folds.

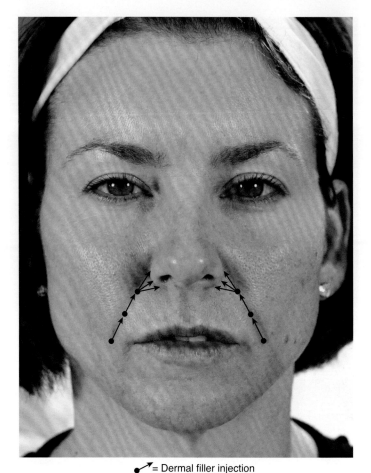

= Dermal filler injection

*FIGURE 3* ● Overview of nasolabial fold dermal filler injections.

- **Cautions**
  - The lateral nasal artery is the main vascular supply for the nasal tip and ala and it is avoided with treatment of the nasolabial folds.
  - The nasolabial fold is a natural facial contour and full effacement can result in an undesirable simian appearance.

## Performing the Procedure: Dermal Filler Treatment of Nasolabial Folds

### Anesthesia

1. Clean and prepare the skin lateral to the nasolabial folds with alcohol.
2. Inject buffered 2% lidocaine-epinephrine solution subcutaneously as shown in Figure 2.
3. Allow a few minutes for anesthesia.

### Dermal Filler

1. Position the patient in a 60-degree reclined position.
2. Prepare the nasolabial folds with alcohol.
3. The provider is positioned on the same side as the nasolabial fold to be injected.

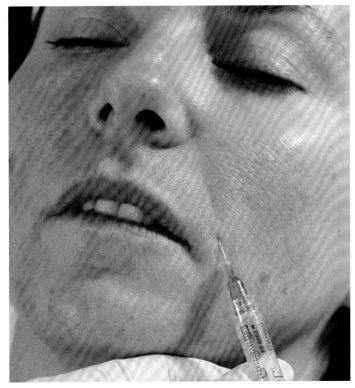

FIGURE 4  ●  First injection for nasolabial fold dermal filler treatment.

4. Attach a 30-gauge, ½-inch needle to the prefilled HA-lidocaine dermal filler syringe. Ensure that the needle is firmly affixed to the dermal filler syringe to prevent the needle popping off when plunger pressure is applied.

5. Prime the needle by depressing the syringe plunger until a small amount of dermal filler extrudes from the needle tip.

6. The first injection point is medial to the nasolabial fold at the inferior portion of the fold (Fig. 4). Insert the needle at a 30-degree angle to the skin, directing it toward the ala, and advance to the needle hub. Apply firm and constant pressure on the syringe plunger, while gradually withdrawing the needle to inject a linear thread of filler in the mid- to deep dermis.

7. The second injection point is approximately 1 cm superior to the first injection point and placed as above (Fig. 5).

8. The third injection point is 1 cm superior to the second injection point and the fanning technique is used. Insert the needle at a 30-degree angle to the skin and advance until the tip lies at the edge of the ala. Inject filler in a linear thread as described above. Without fully withdrawing the needle from the skin, redirect the needle inferiorly and medially using small angulations to ensure dermal filler placement is contiguous (Figs. 6A and 6B). Repeat until desired correction is achieved.

9. Compress the treatment area with thumb on the skin and first finger intraorally to smooth any visible or palpable bumps of filler product. If bumps do not easily compress, the area may be moistened with water and stretched between the provider's fingers. Additional swelling and bruising commonly occur after compression and manipulation of filler product.

10. Repeat the above injections for the contralateral side of the face.

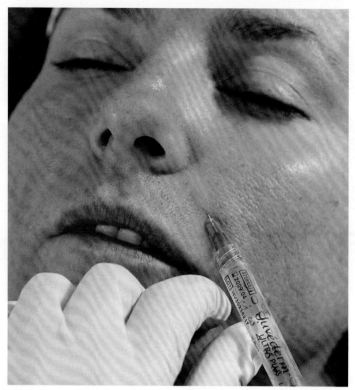

*FIGURE 5* ● Second injection for nasolabial fold dermal filler treatment.

### Tips

- Avoid placing filler product in the superficial dermis as this may result in an undesirable visible ridge of filler, which does not readily compress.
- Avoid treating lateral to the nasolabial folds as this can exacerbate the folds.
- Watch for tissue blanching of the nasal ala and other ischemic signs or symptoms. If ischemia occurs, manage as described in the Complications section.

## Results

- Reduction of nasolabial folds is immediately evident at the time of treatment. Figure 1 shows a 38-year-old woman with moderate nasolabial folds before (A) and 1 week after (B) treatment with 1.6-mL HA dermal filler, Juvederm Ultra Plus.

## Duration of Effects and Subsequent Treatments

- Visible correction of nasolabial folds typically lasts 9 months to 1 year after treatment.
- Subsequent treatment with dermal filler is recommended when the volume of dermal filler product is visibly diminished and nasolabial folds become more evident, prior to their pretreatment appearance.

## Follow-ups and Management

Patients are assessed 4 weeks after treatment to evaluate for reduction of nasolabial folds. Common issues reported by patients during this time include the following:

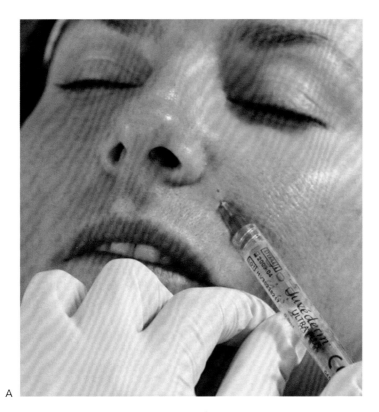

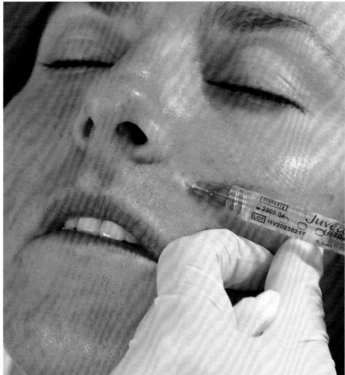

*FIGURE 6* ● Third injection point for nasolabial fold dermal filler treatment **(A)** with medial fanning technique **(B)**.

- **Bruising, swelling, erythema, and tenderness.** See Follow-ups and Management in the Introduction and Foundation Concepts section.
- **Persistent nasolabial folds.** Patients should be assessed for the following:
  - **Static nasolabial folds.** Additional dermal filler may be necessary if a volume deficit persists. Typically 0.4–0.8 mL HA-lidocaine will achieve the desired result.
  - **Dynamic nasolabial folds.** Combination treatment with botulinum toxin may be required to achieve optimal results in patients with deep dynamic nasolabial folds, see Combining Aesthetic Treatments later.

## Complications and Management

- General dermal filler complications and management are reviewed in the Complications section
- Tissue ischemia and tissue necrosis

**Tissue ischemia** resulting from intravascular injection and occlusion of the angular artery may occur with nasolabial fold treatments. Signs of vascular compromise and ischemia include a violaceous reticular pattern or white blanching, and may be painful or painless. These changes may be seen on the nose and/or nasolabial fold, and can present immediately, or be delayed. One case report identified ischemic changes 6 hours after dermal filler treatment. Ischemia is managed urgently as it can rapidly progress to **tissue necrosis** (see Complications section for management).

## Combining Aesthetic Treatments and Maximizing Results

- **Botulinum toxin.** Some patients excessively contract the lip levator muscles during smiling resulting in deep nasolabial folds and a "gummy smile." In these patients, combining dermal filler treatment of the nasolabial fold with botulinum toxin treatment of the levator labii superioris alaeque nasi muscle can improve reduction of nasolabial folds.
- **Dermal filler in adjacent areas.** Patients requiring nasolabial fold treatment may also require treatment of the malar area. Restoring midface volume often reduces nasolabial folds, and it is advisable to perform malar augmentation first and reassess nasolabial folds afterwards (see Malar Augmentation chapter).
- **Dermal filler layering.** Although moderate to severe nasolabial folds can be treated with an HA dermal filler, using the techniques described in this chapter, improved outcomes can often be achieved by layering two types of dermal fillers. Layering is considered an advanced procedure, which consists of placing a dermal filler with more structural support in areas of deep dermal volume loss, and overlaying it with a thinner, more malleable dermal filler to smooth superficial fine lines and wrinkles (see Layering Dermal Fillers chapter).

## Pricing

Dermal filler fees are based on the type of filler used, size and number of syringes, the injector's skill, and vary according to community pricing in different geographic regions. Prices range from $500 to $800 per syringe of 0.8-mL HA for treatment of nasolabial folds.

# Marionette Lines

## Rebecca Small, M.D.

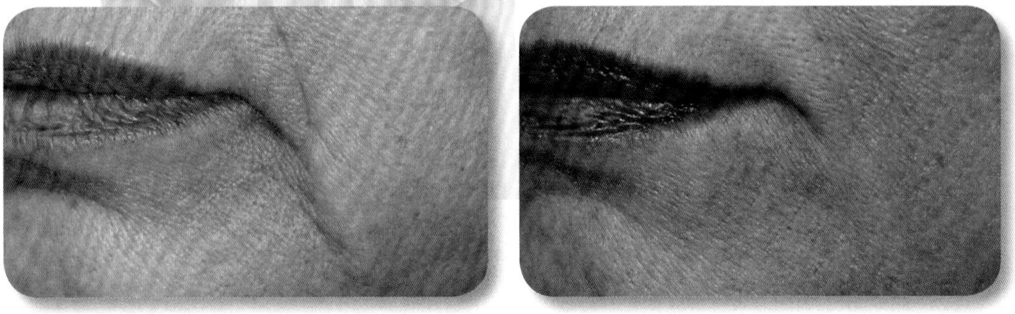

A                      B

*FIGURE 1* ● Marionette lines before **(A)** and 4 weeks after **(B)** dermal filler treatment, using hyaluronic acid.

Prominent marionette lines project sadness, and reduction of these lines is one of the most commonly performed dermal filler procedures. Using appropriate filler volume and injection techniques, support to the lateral lower lip can be restored with correction of marionette lines and downturned oral commissures. In this chapter, reference to marionette lines also includes downturned oral commissures as these often occur together.

## Indications

- Marionette lines
- Downturned oral commissures

## Anatomy

- **Wrinkles, folds, and contours.** The corners of the mouth, where the upper lip meets the lower lip, are called the oral commissures. Marionette lines are folds which descend from the oral commissures toward the jaw (see Dermal Filler Anatomy section, Figs. 1 and 2). Many factors contribute to marionette line formation including soft tissue volume loss and dermal atrophy, biometric volume loss with resorption of mandibular bone, reduced skin elasticity, buccal descent, and hyperdynamic lower face musculature.

## Patient Assessment

- Patients with mild, moderate, and severe static marionette lines are candidates for dermal filler treatments.
- Patients presenting with excess laxity and hanging skin folds usually require surgical intervention for significant improvement.

## Contraindications

- See Contraindications in the Introduction and Foundation Concepts section.

## Treatment Goals

- Reduction of marionette lines with full effacement.
- Repositioning downturned oral commissures to their natural horizontal position.

## Recommended Dermal Filler Product

- Basic hyaluronic acid (HA) dermal filler products that have lidocaine (HA-lidocaine) are recommended for treatment of marionette lines, such as Juvederm® Ultra XC, Juvederm® Ultra Plus XC or Restylane-L® (see Basic and Advanced Procedures in the Introduction and Foundation Concepts section).
- This chapter describes treatment of marionette lines with Juvederm Ultra Plus XC (HA-lidocaine).

## Dermal Filler Treatment Volumes

- The estimated HA dermal filler volume necessary for treatment is based on the patient's observed facial anatomy and volume loss in the treatment area. The following are recommended starting volumes, using HA-lidocaine products:
  - Mild marionette lines typically require 0.8 mL HA-lidocaine.
  - Moderate marionette lines typically require 1.6 mL HA-lidocaine.
  - Severe marionette lines typically require 2.4 mL HA-lidocaine.

## Equipment for Anesthesia

- Local infiltration injection supplies (see Equipment for Injectable Anesthetics in the Anesthesia section)
- Lidocaine HCl 2% with epinephrine 1:100,000 buffered (referred to as buffered 2% lidocaine-epinephrine solution)
- 30-gauge, ½-inch needle

## Equipment for Dermal Filler Procedure

- General dermal filler injection supplies (see Equipment in the Introduction and Foundation Concepts section)
- 30-gauge, ½-inch needle

## Anesthesia Overview

- **Local lidocaine infiltration.** Buffered 2% lidocaine-epinephrine solution can be used to achieve anesthesia for marionette lines.

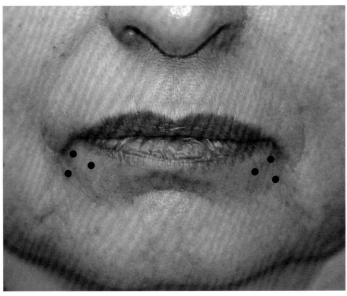

● = 0.1 mL Lidocaine

*FIGURE 2* ● Anesthesia for marionette line dermal filler treatment.

- Both lines are anesthetized using six injections of 0.1 mL for a total volume of 0.6 mL (Fig. 2).
- See Injectable Anesthetics in the Anesthesia section for additional information on local infiltration methods.
- Sensitivity increases with proximity to the lip and injections are started at the inferior portion of the marionette lines.
- **Topical anesthetic.** Benzocaine:lidocaine:tetracaine (BLT) may be used as an alternative for patients with high pain thresholds (see Topical Anesthetics in the Anesthesia section).

## Dermal Filler Procedure Overview

- **Overview.** Two injection techniques are commonly used for treatment of marionette lines (see Techniques for Dermal Filler Injection in the Introduction and Foundation Concepts section):
    - **Fanning technique** is shown in Figure 3 for treatment of marionette lines, and this technique is demonstrated in this chapter.
    - **Cross-hatching technique** is shown in Figure 4 for treatment of marionette lines.
- **Number of injections.** There are one to three medial fanning injections per side depending on the length of the marionette line. Long marionette lines (Fig. 3), require three medial fanning injections whereas short lines may only require one medial fanning injection. The superior most medial fanning injection near the lip is overlaid by a lateral fanning injection. All injections are placed medial to the marionette lines.
- **Injection depth.** Dermal filler is injected in the mid- to deep dermis for treatment of marionette lines.
- **Cautions**
    - Overtreatment can result in undesirable contour changes of the lateral upper lip.
    - Overfilling the marionette line area with dermal filler can result in vascular compromise and possible necrosis.

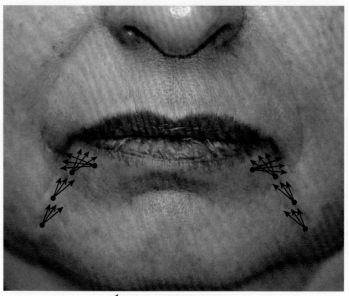

✒ = Dermal filler injection

*FIGURE 3* ● Fanning technique for dermal filler treatment of marionette lines.

## Performing the Procedure: Dermal Filler Treatment of Marionette Lines

### Anesthesia

1. Clean and prepare the skin in the marionette line area with alcohol.
2. Inject buffered lidocaine-epinephrine solution subcutaneously as shown in Figure 2.
3. Allow a few minutes for anesthesia.

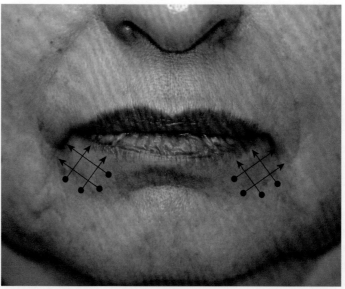

✒ = Dermal filler injection

*FIGURE 4* ● Cross-hatching technique for dermal filler treatment of marionette lines.

## Dermal Filler

1. Position the patient at a 60 degree reclined position.
2. Prepare the marionette line area with alcohol.
3. The provider is positioned on the same side as the marionette line to be injected.
4. Attach a 30-gauge, ½-inch needle to the prefilled HA-lidocaine dermal filler syringe. Ensure that the needle is firmly affixed to the dermal filler syringe to prevent the needle popping off when plunger pressure is applied.
5. Prime the needle by depressing the syringe plunger until a small amount of dermal filler extrudes from the needle tip.
6. The first medial fanning injection is at the inferior portion of the marionette line. Determine the injection point by laying the needle on the skin, parallel and just medial to the marionette line, such that the needle tip is 1 mm below lower lip. The injection point is at the needle hub (Fig. 5A).
7. Insert the needle at a 30-degree angle to the skin, direct it superiorly toward the lip and advance to the needle hub. Apply firm and constant pressure on the syringe plunger while gradually withdrawing needle to inject a linear thread of filler in the mid- to deep dermis. Without fully withdrawing the needle from the skin, redirect the needle medially using small angulations, advance the needle to the hub again and repeat until desired correction is achieved. Ensure dermal filler placement is contiguous. This is referred to as medial fanning (Figs. 5B, 5C, and 5D).
8. The second medial fanning injection is approximately 1 cm inferior to the first injection and placed as described above.
9. The third medial fanning injection is approximately 1 cm inferior to the second injection and placed as described above.
10. The lateral fanning injection is placed just below the border of the lower lip. Determine the injection point by laying the needle on the skin, parallel and just inferior to the lower lip, such that the needle tip is 1 mm medial to the marionette line. The injection point is at the needle hub (Fig. 6A).
11. Insert the needle at a 30-degree angle to the skin, direct it laterally toward the corner of the lips, advanced to the needle hub and fan inferiorly (Figs. 6B and 6C).
12. Compress the treatment area with the thumb on the skin and first finger intraorally, to smooth any visible or palpable bumps of filler product. If bumps do not easily compress, the area may be moistened with water and stretched between the provider's fingers. Additional swelling and bruising commonly occur after compression and manipulation of filler product.
13. Repeat the above injections for the contralateral side of the face.

## Tips

- Avoid placing filler product in the superficial dermis as this may result in an undesirable visible ridge of filler, which does not readily compress.
- Avoid treating lateral to the marionette lines as this can accentuate marionette lines.
- Watch for tissue blanching. If ischemia occurs, manage as described in the Complications section.

## Results

- Reduction of marionette lines is immediately evident at the time of treatment. Figure 1 shows a 69-year-old woman with moderate marionette lines before (A) and 4 weeks after (B) treatment with 1.6-mL HA-lidocaine filler, Juvederm Ultra Plus XC.

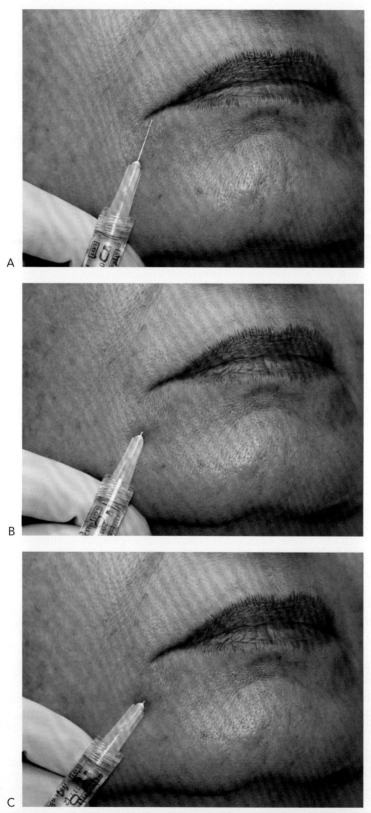

*FIGURE 5* ● Medial fanning for marionette lines dermal filler treatment: needle insertion point determination **(A)** and injection technique **(B, C, D)**.

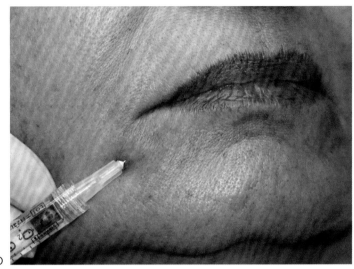

D

*FIGURE 5* (Continued)

## Duration of Effects and Subsequent Treatments

- Visible correction of marionette lines typically lasts 9 months to 1 year after treatment.
- Subsequent treatment with dermal filler is recommended when the volume of dermal filler product is visibly diminished and the marionette lines become more evident, prior to their pretreatment appearance.

## Follow-ups and Management

Patients are assessed 4 weeks after treatment to evaluate for reduction of marionette lines. Common issues reported by patients during this time include the following:

- **Bruising, swelling, erythema, and tenderness.** See Follow-ups and Management in the Introduction and Foundation Concepts section.
- **Persistent marionette lines.** Patients should be assessed for the following:
  - **Static marionette lines.** Additional dermal filler may be necessary if a volume deficit persists. Typically 0.4–0.8 mL HA-lidocaine will achieve the desired result.
  - **Dynamic marionette lines.** Combination treatment with botulinum toxin may be required to achieve optimal results in patients with dynamic marionette lines, see Combining Aesthetic Treatments below.

## Complications and Management

- General dermal filler complications and management are reviewed in the Complications section
- Ischemia and tissue necrosis

   **Ischemia** in the marionette line area is typically due to overfilling the tissue rather than vascular occlusion. It usually presents painlessly, and is visible as immediate blanching. Ischemia is managed urgently as it can rapidly progress to **tissue necrosis**.

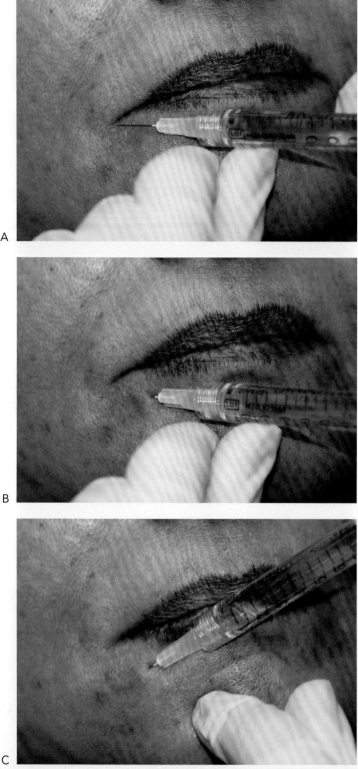

A

B

C

FIGURE 6 ● Lateral fanning for mental crease dermal filler treatment: injection point determination **(A)** and injection technique **(B, C)**.

In the marionette line area this can usually be managed by discontinuing injection and firmly massaging the blanched tissue with the first finger inside the mouth and thumb on the skin. Discontinue massage once the tissue is pink. Further management strategies are discussed in the Complications section. Modify the postprocedure patient instructions, to avoid icing the area that had vascular compromise.

## Combining Aesthetic Treatments and Maximizing Results

- **Botulinum toxin.** Some patients excessively contract the depressor anguli oris muscles which contribute to formation of marionette lines. Combining dermal filler treatment of marionette lines with botulinum toxin treatment of the depressor anguli oris muscles can improve reduction of marionette lines.
- **Dermal filler in adjacent areas.** Patients requiring marionette line dermal filler treatment may also require treatment of the extended mental crease area. If this adjacent area has a volume deficit, concurrent treatment with the marionette lines can enhance results (see Extended Mental Crease chapter).
- **Dermal filler layering.** Although moderate to severe marionette lines can be treated with an HA dermal filler, using the techniques described in this chapter, improved outcomes can often be achieved by layering two types of dermal fillers. Layering is considered an advanced procedure, which consists of placing a dermal filler with more structural support in areas of deep dermal volume loss, and overlaying it with a thinner, more malleable dermal filler to smooth superficial fine lines and wrinkles (see Layering Dermal Fillers chapter).

## Pricing

Dermal filler fees are based on the type of filler used, size and number of syringes, the injector's skill, and vary according to community pricing in different geographic regions. Prices range from $500 to $800 per syringe of 0.8 mL HA for treatment of marionette lines.

# Chapter 3

# Mental Crease

### Rebecca Small, M.D.

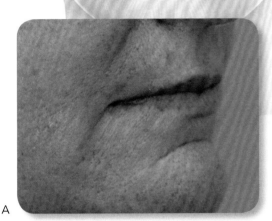 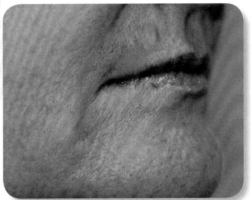

A                                                                                            B

**FIGURE 1** ● Mental crease before **(A)** and 4 weeks after **(B)** dermal filler treatment, using hyaluronic acid.

The mental crease can become more prominent with lower face aging, and dermal filler treatment is frequently performed for the reduction of this crease.

## Indications

• Mental crease

## Anatomy

• **Wrinkles, folds, and contours.** The mental crease, or labiomental crease, is a horizontal line just above the chin (see Dermal Filler Anatomy section, Figs. 1 and 2). Mental crease formation is due to many factors including soft tissue volume loss and dermal atrophy, reduced skin elasticity, biometric volume loss with resorption of mandibular bone and tooth alveolar processes, and hyperdynamic lower face musculature.

## Patient Assessment

• Patients with mild, moderate, and severe static mental creases are candidates for dermal filler treatments.

## Contraindications

- See Contraindications in the Introduction and Foundation Concepts section.

## Treatment Goals

- Reduction of the mental crease without full effacement to preserve the chin contour.

## Recommended Dermal Filler Product

- Basic hyaluronic acid (HA) dermal filler products that have lidocaine (HA-lidocaine) are recommended for treatment of the mental crease, such as Juvederm® Ultra XC, Juvederm® Ultra Plus XC or Restylane-L® (see Introduction and Foundation Concepts in Basic and Advanced Procedures section).
- This chapter describes treatment of the mental crease with Juvederm Ultra Plus XC (HA-lidocaine).

## Dermal Filler Treatment Volumes

- The estimated HA dermal filler volume necessary for treatment is based on the patient's observed facial anatomy and volume loss in the treatment area. Typical starting volumes are listed as follows:
  - Mild mental creases typically require 0.4 mL HA-lidocaine.
  - Moderate to severe mental creases typically require 0.8 mL HA-lidocaine.

## Equipment for Anesthesia

- Local infiltration injection supplies (see Equipment for Injectable Anesthetics in the Anesthesia section)
- Lidocaine HCl 2% with epinephrine 1:100,000 buffered (referred to as buffered 2% lidocaine-epinephrine solution)
- 30-gauge, ½-inch needle

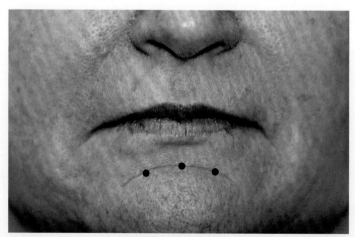

● = 0.1 mL Lidocaine

*FIGURE 2* ● Anesthesia for mental crease dermal filler treatment.

# Equipment for Dermal Filler Procedure

- General dermal filler injection supplies (see Equipment in the Introduction and Foundation Concepts section)
- Lidocaine HCl 2% with epinephrine 1:100,000 (referred to as buffered 2% lidocaine-epinephrine solution)
- 30-gauge, ½-inch needle

# Anesthesia Overview

- **Local lidocaine infiltration.** Buffered 2% lidocaine-epinephrine solution can be used to achieve anesthesia for nasolabial folds.
- The mental crease is anesthetized using three injections of 0.1 mL for a total volume of 0.3 mL (Fig. 2). See Injectable Anesthetics in the Anesthesia section for additional information on local infiltration methods. Sensitivity increases toward the midline of the face, and injections are started at the lateral portion of the crease.
- **Topical anesthetic.** Benzocaine:lidocaine:tetracaine (BLT) may be used as an alternative for patients with high pain thresholds (see Topical Anesthetics in the Anesthesia section).

# Dermal Filler Procedure Overview

- **Overview.** An overview of injection points and injection techinque for treatment of the mental crease using a HA dermal filler is shown in Figure 3.
- **Number of injections.** There are three linear thread injections (see Techniques for Dermal Filler Injection in the Introduction and Foundation Concepts section). Injections start at the lateral most portion of the mental crease and proceed medially.
- **Injection depth.** Dermal filler is injected in the mid- to deep dermis for treatment of the mental crease.
- **Cautions.** This area is not notable for major cautions.

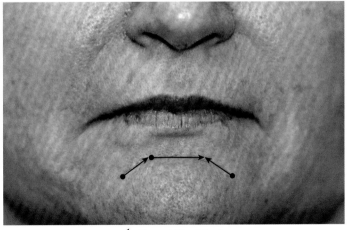

✒ = Dermal filler injection

*FIGURE 3* ● Overview of mental crease dermal filler injections.

## Performing the Procedure: Dermal Filler Treatment of the Mental Crease

### Anesthesia

1. Clean and prepare the skin in the mental crease area with alcohol.
2. Inject buffered 2% lidocaine-epinephrine solution subcutaneously as shown in Figure 2.
3. Allow a few minutes for anesthesia.

### Dermal Filler

1. Position the patient in a 60-degree reclined position.
2. Clean and prepare the skin of the mental crease area with alcohol.
3. The provider is positioned on the same side as the mental crease to be injected.
4. Attach a 30-gauge, ½-inch needle to the prefilled HA-lidocaine dermal filler syringe. Ensure that the needle is firmly affixed to the dermal filler syringe to prevent the needle popping off when plunger pressure is applied.
5. Prime the needle by depressing the syringe plunger until a small amount of dermal filler extrudes from the needle tip.
6. The first injection point is at the inferior lateral portion of the mental crease. Determine the first injection point by laying the needle on top of the skin such that the tip is at one end of the horizontal mental crease. The injection point is at the needle hub (Fig. 4A).
7. Insert the needle at a 30-degree angle to the skin, directing it superiorly and medially following the contour of the mental crease and advance to the needle hub. Apply firm and constant pressure on the syringe plunger while gradually withdrawing needle to inject a linear thread of filler in the mid- to deep dermis (Fig. 4B).
8. The second injection point is approximately 1 cm superior and medial to the first injection point and filler is placed as above, using the linear thread technique to treat the center portion of the mental crease (Fig. 5).
9. Reposition to the opposite side of the patient for the remaining injection.
10. The third injection point is on the opposite side of the mental crease at the inferior lateral portion. The needle is directed superiorly and medially following the contour of the mental crease and filler is placed as above, using the linear thread technique (Fig. 6).
11. Compress the treatment area using both thumbs on the skin and apply firm pressure from medial to lateral, to smooth any visible or palpable bumps of filler product.

## Results

- Reduction of the mental crease is immediately evident at the time of treatment. Figure 1 shows a 47-year-old woman with a moderate mental crease before (A) and 4 weeks after (B) treatment with 0.8-mL HA dermal filler, Juvederm Ultra Plus.

## Duration of Effects and Subsequent Treatments

- Visible correction of the mental crease typically lasts 9 months to 1 year after treatment.
- Subsequent treatment with dermal filler is recommended when the volume of dermal filler product is visibly diminished and the mental crease becomes more evident, prior to the pretreatment appearance.

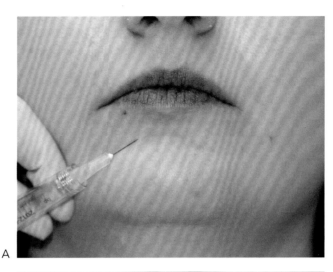

A

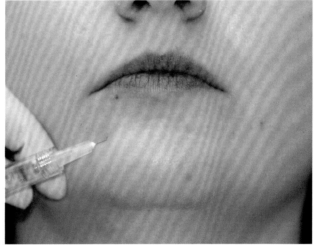

FIGURE 4 ● First injection for mental crease dermal filler treatment: injection point determination (**A**) and threading technique (**B**).

B

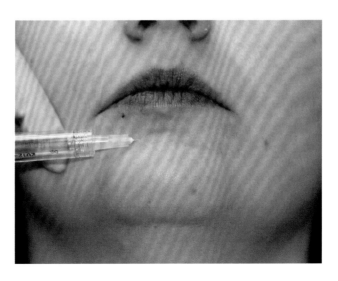

FIGURE 5 ● Second injection for mental crease dermal filler treatment.

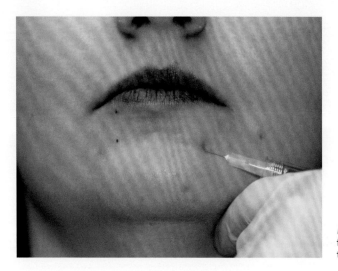

*FIGURE 6* ● Third injection for mental crease dermal filler treatment.

## Follow-ups and Management

Patients are assessed 4 weeks after treatment to evaluate for reduction of the mental crease. Common issues reported by patients during this time include the following:

- **Bruising, swelling, erythema, and tenderness.** See Follow-ups and Management in the Introduction and Foundation Concepts section for recommendations and management strategies.
- **Persistent mental crease.** Patients should be assessed for the following:
  - **Static mental crease.** Additional dermal filler may be necessary if a volume deficit persists. Typically 0.4 mL HA-lidocaine will achieve the desired result.
  - **Dynamic mental crease.** Combination treatment with botulinum toxin may be required to achieve optimal results for a deep mental crease in patients with hyper-dynamic mentalis muscles, see Combining Aesthetic Treatments below.

## Complications and Management

- General dermal filler complications and management are reviewed the Complications section.

## Combining Aesthetic Treatments and Maximizing Results

- **Botulinum toxin.** Some patients have excessive contraction of the mentalis muscle resulting in a deep mental crease. Combining dermal filler treatment of the mental crease with botulinum toxin treatment of the mentalis muscle can improve reduction of the mental crease in these patients.
- **Dermal filler in adjacent areas.** Patients requiring mental crease treatment may also require treatment of the extended mental crease and/or chin areas. If these adjacent areas have volume deficits, concurrent treatment with the mental crease can enhance results (see Extended Mental Crease and Chin Augmentation chapters).

- **Dermal filler layering.** Although moderate to severe mental creases can be treated with an HA dermal filler using the techniques described in this chapter, improved outcomes can often be achieved by layering two types of dermal fillers. Layering is considered an advanced procedure, which consists of placing a dermal filler with more structural support in areas of deep dermal volume loss and overlaying it with a thinner, more malleable dermal filler to smooth superficial fine lines and wrinkles (see Layering chapter).

## Pricing

Dermal filler fees are based on the type of filler used, size and number of syringes, the injector's skill, and vary according to community pricing in different geographic regions. Prices range from $500 to $800 per syringe of 0.8 mL HA for treatment of the mental crease.

# Chapter 4

# Extended Mental Creases

Rebecca Small, M.D.

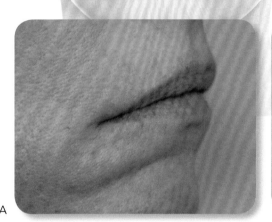 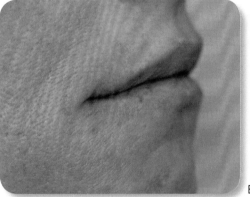

A      B

**FIGURE 1** ● Extended mental crease lateral view before **(A)** and 4 weeks after **(B)** dermal filler treatment using calcium hydroxylapatite.

Extended mental creases can become visible with aging of the lower face, and project sadness or a dour appearance. This area exhibits deep volume loss and correction is achieved with dermal filler products that offer more structural support. Therefore, reduction of the extended mental crease is considered an advanced dermal filler procedure.

## Indications

- Extended mental creases

## Anatomy

- **Wrinkles, folds, and contours.** The extended mental crease is a triangular shaped area of volume loss that lies inferior to the oral commissure. It is bounded laterally by the marionette line, medially by the mental crease, and inferiorly by the chin (Fig. 2A) (see Dermal Filler Anatomy section, Figs. 1 and 2). Extended mental crease formation results from many factors, including soft-tissue volume loss, dermal atrophy, and biometric volume loss due to resorption of mandibular bone and tooth alveolar processes.

85

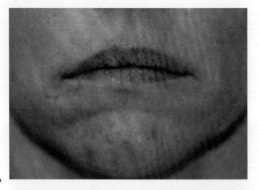

A

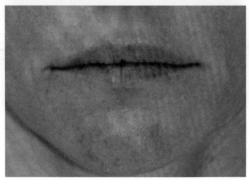

B

*FIGURE 2* ● Extended mental crease front view before **(A)** and 4 weeks after **(B)** dermal filler treatment using calcium hydroxylapatite.

## Patient Assessment

- Patients with mild, moderate, and severe extended mental creases are candidates for dermal filler treatments.

## Contraindications

- See Contraindications in the Introduction and Foundation Concepts section.

## Treatment Goals

- Full effacement of extended mental creases.

## Recommended Dermal Filler Product

- This is an area of deep volume loss and is ideally treated with advanced dermal filler products that offer more structural support, such as Radiesse® (calcium hydroxylapatite [CaHA]), or Perlane-L® (hyaluronic acid [HA]). Juvederm® Ultra Plus, one of the basic HA filler products, provides moderate structural support and can also be used (see Basic and Advanced Procedures in the Introduction and Foundation Concepts section).
- This chapter describes treatment of extended mental creases with CaHA (Radiesse), in particular CaHA that has been mixed with a small amount of lidocaine (CaHA-lidocaine). CaHA-lidocaine has reduced viscosity and a mild anesthetic effect (See Calcium Hydroxylapatite and Lidocaine Preparation in the Introduction and Foundation Concepts section).

## Dermal Filler Treatment Volumes

- The estimated CaHA-lidocaine (Radiesse) dermal filler volume necessary for treatment is based on the patient's observed facial anatomy and volume loss in the treatment area. Typical starting volumes are listed as follows:
  - Mild extended mental creases typically require a total volume of 0.8-mL CaHA-lidocaine.
  - Moderate-to-severe extended mental creases typically require a total volume of 1.6-mL CaHA-lidocaine.

## Equipment for Anesthesia

- Local infiltration injection supplies (see Equipment for Injectable Anesthetics in the Anesthesia section)
- Lidocaine HCl 2% with epinephrine 1:100,000 buffered (referred to as buffered 2% lidocaine-epinephrine solution)
- 30-gauge, ½-inch needle

## Equipment for Dermal Filler Procedure

- General dermal filler injection supplies (see Equipment in the Introduction and Foundation Concepts section)
- 27-gauge, 1¼-inch needle

## Anesthesia Overview

- **Local lidocaine infiltration.** Buffered 2% lidocaine-epinephrine solution can be used to achieve anesthesia for nasolabial folds. The extended mental crease is anesthetized using six injections of 0.1 mL for a total volume of 0.6 mL (Fig. 3). See Injectable Anesthetics in the Anesthesia section for additional information on local infiltration methods. Sensitivity increases with proximity to the lip, and injections are started at the lateral portion of the crease.

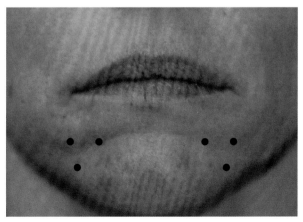

● = 0.1 mL Lidocaine

FIGURE 3　●　Anesthesia for extended mental crease dermal filler treatment.

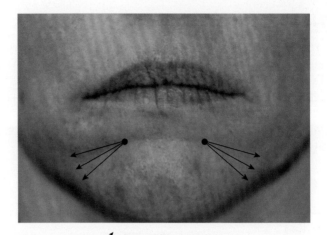

= Dermal filler injection

**FIGURE 4** ● Overview of extended mental crease dermal filler injections.

## Dermal Filler Procedure Overview

- **Overview.** An overview of injection points and injection technique for treatment of the extended mental crease using CaHA-lidocaine dermal filler is shown in Figure 4.
- **Number of injections.** One injection per side is administered using the fanning technique, angulating superiorly (see Techniques for Dermal Filler Injection in the Introduction and Foundation Concepts section).
- **Injection depth.** Dermal filler is injected in the deep dermis for treatment of the extended mental creases.
- **Cautions.** This area is not notable for major cautions.

## Performing the Procedure: Dermal Filler Treatment of Extended Mental Crease

### Anesthesia

1. Clean and prepare the skin in the extended mental crease area with alcohol.
2. Inject buffered 2% lidocaine-epinephrine solution subcutaneously as shown in Figure 3.
3. Allow a few minutes for anesthesia.

### Dermal Filler

1. Position the patient in a 60-degree reclined position.
2. Clean and prepare the skin of the mental crease area with alcohol.
3. The provider is positioned on the opposite side of the extended mental crease to be injected.
4. Attach a 27-gauge, 1¼-inch needle to the CaHA-lidocaine dermal filler syringe. Ensure that the needle is firmly affixed to the dermal filler syringe to prevent the needle from popping off when plunger pressure is applied.
5. Prime the needle by depressing the syringe plunger until a small amount of dermal filler extrudes from the needle tip.
6. The injection point is at the medial portion of the extended mental crease where it approaches the lateral edge of the mental crease. Determine the first injection point

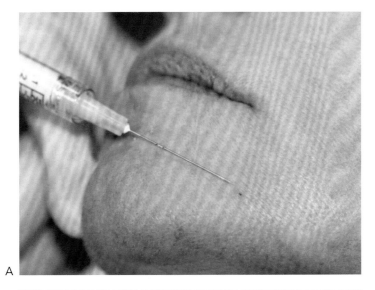

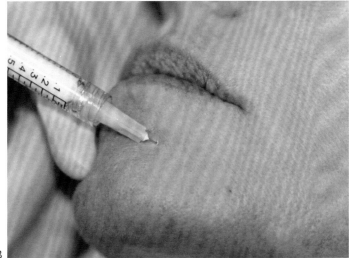

FIGURE 5 ● Extended mental crease dermal filler treatment: needle insertion point determination **(A)** and injection technique **(B)**.

by laying the needle above the skin such that the needle hub is at the lateral mental crease. The injection point is at the needle hub (Fig. 5A).

7. Insert the needle at a 30-degree angle to the skin, directing it laterally toward the marionette line, and advance to the needle hub (Fig. 5B). Apply firm and constant pressure on the syringe plunger while gradually withdrawing the needle to inject a linear thread of filler in the deep dermis. Fan the needle inferiorly without fully withdrawing the needle from the skin using small angulations to ensure dermal filler placement is contiguous. Repeat until desired correction is achieved.

8. Reposition to the opposite side of the patient for the remaining injection and repeat as above.

9. Compress the treatment areas using both thumbs on the skin and apply firm pressure from medial to lateral, to smooth any visible or palpable bumps of the filler.

## Tip

- Avoid placing filler too superficially as dermal filler products with more structural support can be seen as visible bumps.

## Results

- Reduction of the extended mental crease is immediately evident at the time of treatment. Figures 1 and 2 show a 48-year-old woman with a moderate-to-severe extended mental crease before (A) and 4 weeks after (B) treatment with 1.4 mL of a CaHA-lidocaine dermal filler, Radiesse.

## Duration of Effects and Subsequent Treatments

- Visible correction of the extended mental crease treated with CaHA-lidocaine typically lasts for 1–1½ years.
- Subsequent treatment with the dermal filler is recommended when the volume of the dermal filler product is visibly diminished and the extended mental creases become more evident, prior to their pretreatment appearance.

## Follow-ups and Management

Patients are assessed 4 weeks after treatment to evaluate for reduction of the mental crease. Common issues reported by patients during this time include:

- **Bruising, swelling, erythema, and tenderness.** See Follow-ups and Management in the Introduction and Foundation Concepts section for recommendations and management strategies.
- **Persistent extended mental crease.** Additional dermal filler may be necessary if a volume deficit persists. Typically 0.3–0.4 mL CaHA-lidocaine will achieve the desired result. If possible, use ice or topical anesthetic with touch-up to reduce tissue distortion that can occur with local lidocaine injection.

## Complications and Management

- General dermal filler complications and management are reviewed in Complications section.

## Combining Aesthetic Treatments and Maximizing Results

- **Dermal filler in adjacent areas.** Patients requiring extended mental crease treatment may also have volume deficits in the mental crease, chin, and/or marionette line areas. If these adjacent areas have volume deficits, concurrent treatment of the extended mental crease may enhance results (see Mental Crease, Chin Augmentation, and Marionette Line chapters).

## Pricing

Dermal filler fees are based on the type of filler used, size and number of syringes, the injector's skill, and vary according to community pricing in different geographic regions. Prices range from $550 to $900 per syringe of 0.8 mL CaHA (Radiesse) for treatment of the extended mental crease.

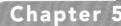

# Chin Augmentation

Rebecca Small, M.D.

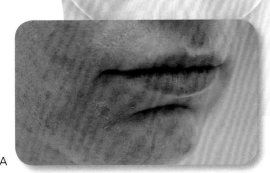
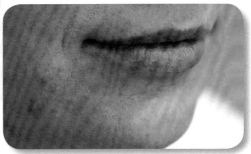

A                        B

**FIGURE 1** ● Recessed chin before **(A)** and 4 weeks after **(B)** dermal filler chin augmentation treatment, using calcium hydroxylapatite.

Treatment of a recessed chin has traditionally been a surgical procedure utilizing chin implants. This undesirable contour can also be effectively treated with dermal fillers. Products which offer more structural support to the tissues are used for chin augmentation and this is, therefore, considered an advanced dermal filler procedure.

## Indications

- Recessed, flat chin

## Anatomy

- **Wrinkles, folds, and contour changes.** Two basic chin shapes can be seen from the anterior view: triangular (Fig. 2A) and square (Fig. 2B). Typically, men have square-shaped chins and women have triangular chins. However, both shapes can be seen in either gender and can exhibit undesirable recessed or flattened contours.

## Patient Assessment

- Chin projection is assessed from the anterior and lateral views. In profile, the anterior-most projection of the chin should be just slightly behind the anterior projection of the lower lip. The chin should appear rounded and not flat.

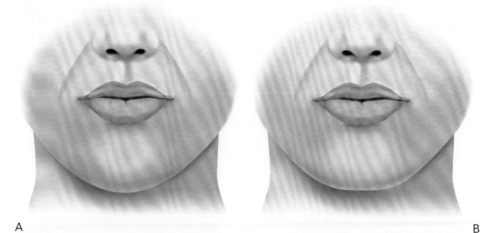

A                                                                                                  B

*FIGURE 2* ● Triangular **(A)** and square **(B)** chin shapes.

- Dermal filler chin augmentation is indicated for a recessed or flattened chin due to soft-tissue changes, but not for dental and skeletal conditions, such as excessive overbite or micrognathia. Excessive overbite can be assessed by having the patient bite down and observing the dentition for malocclusion.

## Contraindications

- See Contraindications in the Introduction and Foundation Concepts section.
- Very small or severely recessed chins seen with conditions such as micrognathia, severe malocclusion, and craniofacial abnormalities.

## Treatment Goals

- Increased anterior projection and rounding of the chin.

## Recommended Dermal Filler Product

- This is an area of deep volume loss and is ideally treated with advanced dermal filler products that offer more structural support, such as Radiesse® (calcium hydroxylapatite [CaHA]) or Perlane-L® (hyaluronic acid [HA]) (see Basic and Advanced Procedures in the Introduction and Foundation Concepts section).
- This chapter describes chin augmentation with CaHA (Radiesse). CaHA is not mixed with lidocaine for maximum structural support.

## Dermal Filler Treatment Volumes

- The estimated CaHA (Radiesse) dermal filler volume necessary for treatment is based on patients' observed facial anatomy and volume loss in the treatment area. Typical starting volumes are listed as follows:
  - Mild chin recession and flattening typically requires a total volume of 0.6–0.8 mL CaHA.

- Moderate-to-severe chin recession and flattening typically requires a total volume of 1.3–1.5 mL CaHA.

## Equipment for Anesthesia

- Local infiltration injection supplies (see Equipment for Injectable Anesthetics in the Anesthesia section)
- Lidocaine HCl 2% with epinephrine 1:100,000 buffered (referred to as buffered 2% lidocaine-epinephrine solution)
- 30-gauge, ½-inch needle
- General topical anesthetic supplies (see Equipment for Topical Anesthetics in the Anesthesia section)
- Benzocaine:lidocaine:tetracaine (BLT) ointment

## Equipment for Dermal Filler Procedure

- General dermal filler injection supplies (see Equipment in the Introduction and Foundation Concepts section)
- 27-gauge, 1¼-inch needle

## Anesthesia Overview

- **Local lidocaine infiltration.** Buffered 2% lidocaine-epinephrine solution can be used to achieve anesthesia for the needle insertion site.
  - **Triangular chin** needle insertion sites are anesthetized using one injection of 0.1 mL buffered 2% lidocaine-epinephrine solution (Fig. 3).
  - **Square chin** needle insertion sites are anesthetized using two injections of 0.1 mL for a total of 0.2 mL buffered 2% lidocaine-epinephrine solution.
- **Topical anesthetic.** BLT is used on the remainder of the chin (see Topical Anesthetics in the Anesthesia section).

## Overview of Dermal Filler Procedure

- **Overview.** Different methods are used to treat triangular versus square-shaped chins. An overview of chin augmentation injection points and injection techniques are shown

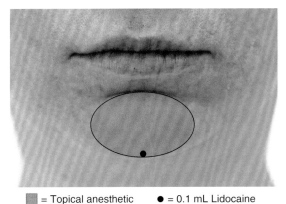

▨ = Topical anesthetic   ● = 0.1 mL Lidocaine

**FIGURE 3** ● Anesthesia for chin augmentation dermal filler treatment.

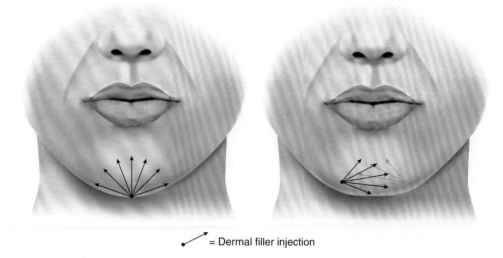

= Dermal filler injection

A                                                                                              B

*FIGURE 4* ● Overview of chin augmentation dermal filler injections for triangular **(A)** and square-shaped **(B)** chins.

for triangular (Fig. 4A) and square-shaped (Fig. 4B) chins. This chapter demonstrates dermal filler injection for a triangular chin.

- **Number of injections.** There are two fanning injections (see Techniques for Dermal Filler Injection in the Introduction and Foundation Concepts section) for a triangular chin.
- **Injection depth.** Dermal filler is injected in the deep dermis for chin augmentation.
- **Cautions.** This area is not notable for major cautions.

## Performing the Procedure: Dermal Filler Chin Augmentation

### Anesthesia

1. Clean and prepare the skin of the chin with alcohol.
2. Inject 0.1 mL buffered 2% lidocaine-epinephrine solution subcutaneously, as shown in Figure 3.
3. Apply 0.5 g BLT in a thin layer over the chin (Fig. 3); occlusion with a plastic wrap is not necessary.
4. Remove BLT 15–30 minutes after application using alcohol.

### Dermal Filler

1. Position the patient in a 45-degree reclined position.
2. Clean and prepare the skin of the chin with alcohol.
3. The provider is positioned on the opposite side of the chin to be injected.
4. Attach a 27-gauge, 1¼-inch needle to the CaHA dermal filler syringe. Ensure that the needle is firmly affixed to the dermal filler syringe to prevent the needle from popping off when plunger pressure is applied.

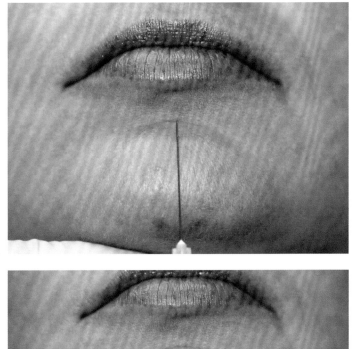

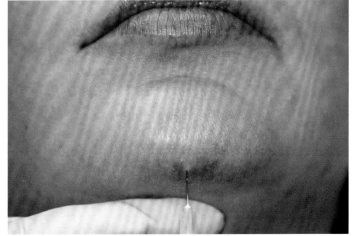

FIGURE 5 ● Dermal filler chin augmentation: needle insertion point determination **(A)** and injection technique **(B)**.

5. Prime the needle by depressing the syringe plunger until a small amount of dermal filler extrudes from the needle tip.
6. The injection point is in the midline just inferior jaw line. Determine the first injection point by laying the needle on top of the chin such that the needle tip reaches the circumference of the chin at the 12 o'clock position. The injection point is at the needle hub (Fig. 5A).
7. Insert the needle and direct it superiorly toward the lower lip at the 12 o'clock position (Fig. 5B). Advance the needle, taking care to follow the curve of the chin. Apply firm and constant pressure on the syringe plunger while gradually withdrawing the needle to inject a linear thread of filler in the deep dermis. When placing dermal filler in the *left* half of the chin, fan the needle *clockwise* without fully withdrawing the needle from the skin, using small angulations to ensure dermal filler placement is contiguous. Continue fanning until the jaw line is reached and then withdraw the needle.
8. Reposition to the opposite side of the patient.

9.  The needle is reinserted at the same injection point in the midline, just inferior the jaw line. When placing dermal filler in the *right* half of the chin, fan the needle *counterclockwise* until the jaw line is reached and then withdraw the needle.
10. Compress the treatment area with both thumbs on the skin using firm pressure from medial to lateral and around the perimeter of the chin, to smooth any visible or palpable bumps of filler.
11. Palpate the treatment area to determine whether there are any skipped areas where filler is not palpable. If necessary, insert the needle at the same injection site and inject linear threads until the desired correction is achieved. Occasionally, a different angle of injection is required to fill skipped areas and the needle can be inserted anywhere in the chin area to achieve confluent filler placement.
12. Compress the treatment area again as described above.

## Tip

- Avoid placing the filler too superficially as dermal filler products with more structural support can be seen as visible bumps.

## Results

- Chin augmentation is immediately evident at the time of treatment. Figure 1 shows a 34-year-old woman with a severely flattened and recessed chin before (A) and 4 weeks after (B) treatment with 1.5 mL of a CaHA dermal filler, Radiesse.

## Duration of Effects and Subsequent Treatments

- Chin augmentation with CaHA typically lasts for 1–1½ years.
- Subsequent treatment with the dermal filler is recommended when the volume of the filler is visibly diminished and the chin contour begins to flatten or become recessed again, prior to the pretreatment appearance.

### Follow-ups and Management

Patients are assessed 4 weeks after treatment to evaluate for adequacy of chin augmentation. Common issues reported by patients include:

- **Bruising, swelling, erythema, and tenderness.** See Follow-ups and Management in the Introduction and Foundation Concepts section for recommendations and management strategies.
- **Asymmetry of the chin.** Additional dermal filler may be necessary if a volume deficit is visible. A typical touch-up procedure requires 0.2–0.3 mL CaHA to address small volume deficits. If possible, use ice or topical anesthetic for anesthesia when performing a touch-up procedure to reduce tissue distortion that can occur with local lidocaine infiltration.

## Complications and Management

- General dermal filler complications and management are reviewed in Complications section.

# Combining Aesthetic Treatments and Maximizing Results

- **Botulinum toxin.** Some patients have excessive contraction of the mentalis muscle, resulting in chin flattening and a deep mental crease. Combining dermal filler chin augmentation with botulinum toxin treatment of the mentalis muscle can improve chin augmentation results in these patients.
- **Dermal filler in adjacent areas.** Patients requiring chin augmentation may also have volume deficits in the mental crease and/or extended mental crease areas. If these adjacent areas have volume deficits, concurrent treatment with chin augmentation can enhance results (see Mental Crease and Extended Mental Crease chapters).

# Pricing

Dermal filler fees are based on the type of filler used, size and number of syringes, the injector's skill, and vary according to community pricing in different geographic regions. Prices range from $650 to $1200 per syringe of 1.5 mL CaHA for chin augmentation.

# Chapter 6

# Lip Border

### Rebecca Small, M.D.

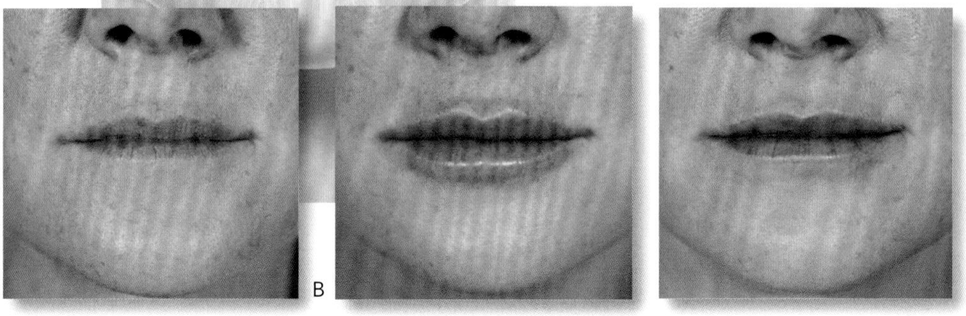

FIGURE 1 ● Lip augmentation before **(A)**, immediately after **(B)**, and 1 week after dermal filler treatment **(C)**, using hyaluronic acid.

Using proper technique and products, dermal filler treatments can enhance lip shape and volume in a natural way. These procedures can benefit patients with less defined lip shape and diminished lip volume from aging; as well as younger patients seeking lip enhancement.

## Indications

- Lip atrophy

## Anatomy

- **Wrinkles, folds, and contours.** The vermillion border is the demarcation between the less keratinized pink vermillion of the lip epidermis, and the highly keratinized facial skin epidermis. The Cupid's bow is the central portion of the upper lip with two peaks at the philtral columns. The Cupid's bow contributes to the natural shape of the lip and is typically enhanced as part of dermal filler lip augmentation (see Dermal Filler Anatomy section, Figs. 1 and 2).

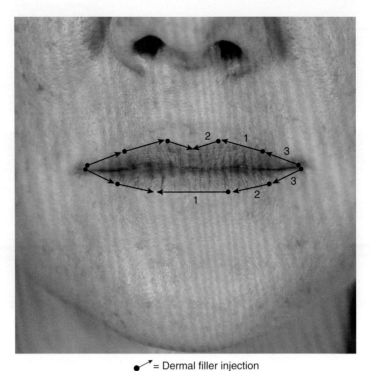

= Dermal filler injection

*FIGURE 2* ● Overview of lip border dermal filler injections.

## Patient Assessment

- Careful consultation and examination using a mirror is necessary to determine lip features that the patient would like enhanced, discuss realistic expectations and advise about aesthetic outcomes. The following points are typically included:
  - A given lip shape can only be enhanced with dermal filler treatment, it cannot be altered into another lip shape.
  - Defining the lip shape and the line around the lips with lip border treatments involves dermal filler placement in the vermillion border.
  - Enhancing the lip body involves placement of dermal filler in the mucosa of the lip.
  - Lip augmentation often combines enhancement of both the lip border and the lip body (see Lip Body chapter).

## Contraindications

- See Contraindications in the Introduction and Foundation Concepts section.
- **Very thin, diminutive upper lip.** Dermal filler treatment of this lip architecture can result in an unnatural anterior projection of the upper lip or a "duck" lip.
- **Braces.** Braces on the teeth can distort lip projection and it is best to avoid dermal filler treatment if they are present.

## Treatment Goals

- Natural fuller appearance to the lip with slight eversion of the vermillion border to enhance lip shape without excessive anterior projection. Lip fullness should be congruent with the patient's age.

# Recommended Dermal Filler Product

- Hyaluronic acid (HA) dermal filler products that have lidocaine (HA-lidocaine) are recommended for treatment of the lip border. Products with a soft tissue filling effect, such as Juvederm® Ultra XC (see Basic and Advanced Procedures in the Introduction and Foundation Concepts section), are recommended for patients with atrophic lips. Products with firmer tissue filling effects, such as Juvederm® Ultra Plus XC and Restylane-L®, are recommended for younger patients (ages 20s–30s) who have greater baseline tissue density and lip volume.
- This chapter describes treatment of the lip border using Juvederm Ultra Plus XC (HA-lidocaine).

# Dermal Filler Treatment Volumes

- The estimated HA dermal filler volume necessary for treatment is based on patients' observed facial anatomy and volume loss in the treatment area.
- Treatment of the upper and lower lip vermillion borders typically requires 0.6–0.8 mL Juvederm Ultra Plus XC, Juvederm Ultra XC, or Restylane-L.

# Equipment for Anesthesia

- Lip ring block supplies (see Equipment for Injectable Anesthetics in the Anesthesia section)
- Lidocaine HCl 2% with epinephrine 1:100,000 buffered or unbuffered (referred to as 2% lidocaine-epinephrine solution)
- 30-gauge, ½-inch needle

# Equipment for Dermal Filler Procedure

- General dermal filler injection supplies (see Equipment in the Introduction and Foundation Concepts section)
- 30-gauge, ½-inch needle

# Anesthesia Overview

- **Lip ring block.** Adequate anesthesia of the lip prior to dermal filler injection is essential for successful lip border treatments. Patients usually require profound lip anesthesia. Dermal fillers formulated or mixed with lidocaine do not offer sufficient pain control for lip filler treatments and a lip ring block is required (see Lip Ring Block in the Anesthesia section).

# Dermal Filler Procedure Overview

- **Overview.** An overview of injection points and injection technique for dermal filler treatment of the lip border shown in Figure 2.
- **Number of injections.** There are six linear thread injections for the upper lip border and five linear thread injections for the lower lip border—a total of 11 injections (see Techniques for Dermal Filler Injection in the Introduction and Foundation Concepts section).

- **Injection depth.** Dermal filler injections are placed in the superficial dermis of the vermillion border.
- **Cautions**
  - Observe filler volumes closely during treatment and administer equal volumes on both sides of the lips, unless gross asymmetry is present prior to treatment.
  - Lip edema can occur rapidly. At the completion of treatment, the side injected first may appear larger due to edema. If asymmetry is evident at the completion of treatment, and injection volumes and palpable product have been consistent for both sides, then it is advisable to reassess symmetry at the follow-up visit once edema has resolved.
  - Avoid overfilling the lateral portion of the upper lip as this can result in undesired contour changes of the lip.
  - Dermal filler can tract outside of the vermillion border resulting in filler collections outside of the intended treatment area, in either the surrounding skin or to the lip mucosa.

## Performing the Procedure: Dermal Filler Treatment of the Lip Border

### Anesthesia

1. Clean and prepare the lips with alcohol, removing all lipstick if present.
2. Perform a lip ring block (see Ring Block in the Anesthesia section) as follows:
   - For the upper lip, use a total volume of 1.2 mL 2% lidocaine-epinephrine solution.
   - For the lower lip, use a total volume of 1.2 mL 2% lidocaine-epinephrine solution.
   - For the corners of the lips, use a total volume of 0.2 mL 2% lidocaine-epinephrine solution.
3. Wait 3–5 minutes for anesthesia.

### Dermal Filler Upper Lip Border

1. Position the patient in a 60-degree reclined position.
2. Prepare the lips with alcohol.
3. Attach a 30-gauge, ½-inch needle to the prefilled HA-lidocaine dermal filler syringe. Ensure that the needle is firmly affixed to the dermal filler syringe to prevent the needle popping off when plunger pressure is applied.
4. Prime the needle by depressing the syringe plunger until a small amount of dermal filler extrudes from the needle tip.
5. The provider is positioned on the same side as the lip to be injected.
6. Identify the first injection point in the upper lip border by laying the needle against the vermillion border such that the needle tip ends at the ipsilateral peak of the Cupid's bow. The injection point is at the needle hub (Fig. 3A).
7. Insert the needle into the vermillion border at a 30-degree angle to the skin and direct it toward the ipsilateral peak of the Cupid's bow (Fig. 3B). Advance to the hub, then apply firm and constant pressure on the syringe plunger while gradually withdrawing needle to inject a linear thread of filler. The filler should flow easily into the vermillion border and a rolled border to the lip will be visible as the filler product is injected.

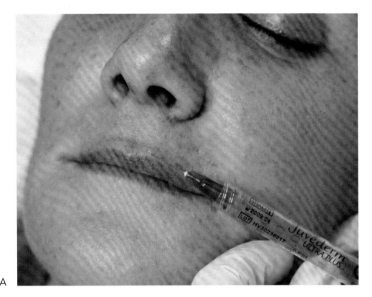

A

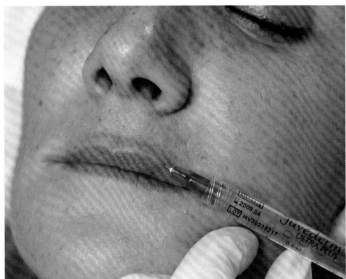

B

FIGURE 3 ● First injection for dermal filler treatment of the upper lip border: needle insertion point determination **(A)** and injection technique **(B)**.

8. The second injection point in the upper lip border is at the ipsilateral peak of the Cupid's bow. Insert the needle and advance inferior-medially to the nadir of the Cupid's bow. Smoothly inject a small amount of filler as the needle is withdrawn (Fig. 4).

9. The third injection point in the upper lip border is one needle length lateral to the first injection point. The needle is inserted until the tip is adjacent to the linear thread from the previous injection, and filler is smoothly injected as the needle is withdrawn (Fig. 5).

10. Gently compress the lip with thumb on the skin and first finger intraorally, and slowly compress from medial to lateral along the length of the lip to smooth any visible or palpable bumps of filler product. If bumps do not easily compress, the area may be

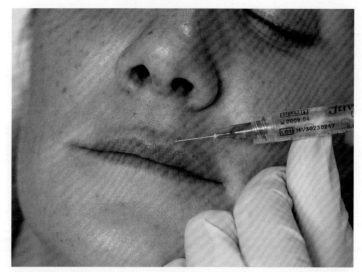

**FIGURE 4** ● Second injection for dermal filler treatment of the upper lip border.

moistened with water and stretched between the provider's fingers. Additional swelling and bruising commonly occur after compression and manipulation of filler product.

11. Reposition to the opposite side of the patient and repeat the above injections for the contralateral upper lip vermillion border.

## Dermal Filler Lower Lip Border

1. Repeat steps 1–5 as above.
2. Identify the first lower lip border injection point by laying the needle against the vermillion border such that the length of the needle spans the center portion of the

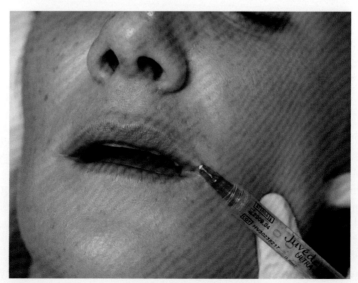

**FIGURE 5** ● Third injection for dermal filler treatment of the upper lip border.

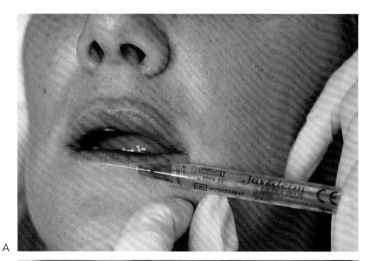

A

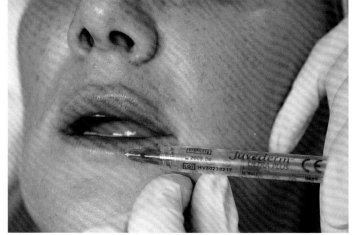

B

*FIGURE 6* ● First injection for dermal filler treatment of the lower lip border: needle insertion point determination **(A)** and injection technique **(B)**.

lower lip; the needle hub is usually just lateral to the ipsilateral peak of the Cupid's bow. The injection point is at the needle hub (Fig 6A).

3. The needle is inserted into the vermillion border at a 30-degree angle to the lip epidermis and directed along the vermillion border toward the opposite side. The needle is advanced to the hub and filler is smoothly injected as the needle is withdrawn (Fig. 6B).

4. The second lower lip border injection point is one needle length lateral to the first injection point. The needle is inserted to the hub and filler is smoothly injected as the needle is withdrawn (Fig. 7).

5. The third lower lip border injection point is at the corner of the lip. The needle is inserted until the tip is adjacent to the linear thread from the previous injection, and filler is smoothly injected as the needle is withdrawn (Fig. 8).

6. Gently compress the lip from medial to lateral as described earlier.

7. Reposition to the opposite side and repeat second and third injections as described earlier for the remainder of the lower lip vermillion border.

8. Proceed with lip body dermal filler injections if also augmenting this area (see Lip Body chapter).

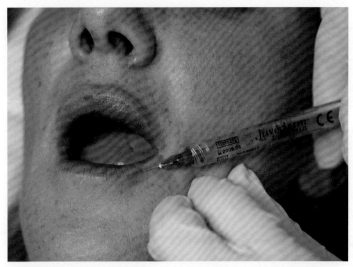

**FIGURE 7** ● Second injection for dermal filler treatment of the lower lip border.

### Tips

- Filler should be smooth and confluent in the vermillion border. If there is a visible or palpable skipped area, inject this area using the above technique until filler product is contiguous and desired correction is achieved.
- If filler is seen outside of the vermillion border during injection, discontinue injection and compress the area until no product is visible outside of the vermillion border and then resume treatment.

## Results

- Lip augmentation is immediately evident at the time of treatment, and there usually is significant edema. Lips may appear overfilled and project anteriorly due to edema. Once edema resolves, lips will appear more defined with improved architecture and fullness

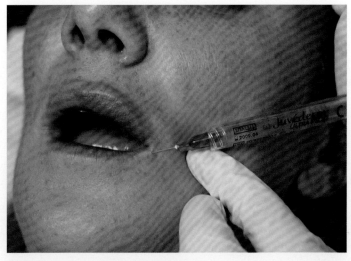

**FIGURE 8** ● Third injection for dermal filler treatment of the lower lip border.

and return to their anatomic position. Figure 1 shows a 38-year-old woman before (A), immediately after (B), and 1 week after (C), lip augmentation with 1.6-mL HA dermal filler, Juvederm Ultra Plus, in the vermillion border and the body of the lips.

## Duration of Effects and Subsequent Treatments

- Lip augmentation typically lasts 6–9 months after treatment as this is a highly mobile region.
- Subsequent treatment with dermal filler is recommended when the volume of dermal filler product is visibly diminished.

## Follow-ups and Management

Patients are assessed 4 weeks after treatment to evaluate for adequacy of lip augmentation and symmetry. Common issues reported by patients include the following:

- **Bruising, swelling, erythema, and tenderness.** See Follow-ups and Management in the Introduction and Foundation Concepts section. Lip edema typically resolves within 3–5 days. Patients often require reassurance to this effect. Application of ice immediately after the procedure and as directed in the aftercare instructions (Appendix 2) can reduce swelling.
- **Mild lip asymmetry.** Asymmetry may be due to too little or too much filler in lip areas.
  - **Additional filler required.** Identify the areas where more filler is desired, both visually and by palpation. The small region requiring a touch-up can be anesthetized using the lip ring block method, by placing lidocaine intraorally adjacent to the region where the touch up is required. The amount necessary for the touch up will vary based on the volume deficit, and it is typically 0.1–0.3 mL HA-lidocaine.
  - **Too much filler or uneven placement.** Small collections of filler can usually be compressed and smoothed. Large collections may require hyaluronidase injection or, as a last resort, incision and expression of product (see Complications section).

## Complications and Management

- General dermal filler complications and management are reviewed in the Complications section
- Swelling and bruising
- Oral herpes simplex reactivation

**Significant swelling and bruising** are the most common side effects with lip augmentation dermal filler treatments (see Complications section, and Follow-ups and Management in the Introduction and Foundation Concepts section).

**Reactivation of oral herpes simplex** is not uncommon and prophylactic antiviral therapy typically suppresses reactivation (see Preprocedure Checklist in the Introduction and Foundation Concepts section).

## Combining Aesthetic Treatments and Maximizing Results

- **Botulinum toxin.** The orbicularis oris muscle which encircles the mouth, functions to pucker lips and invert the vermillion border, and overtime, this can contribute to reduced lip volume and radial lip line formation. Botulinum toxin treatment of the orbicularis oris muscle is commonly used adjunctively with dermal fillers for lip augmentation, as it everts the lips slightly and enhances lip fullness.

- **Dermal filler in adjacent areas.** Enhanced lip fullness can be achieved with concurrent dermal filler treatment of the lip border and lip body (see Lip Body chapter).

## Pricing

Dermal filler fees are based on the type of filler used, size and number of syringes, injector's skill, and vary according to community pricing in different geographic regions. Prices range from $500 to $800 per syringe of 0.8 mL HA for lip augmentation treatment.

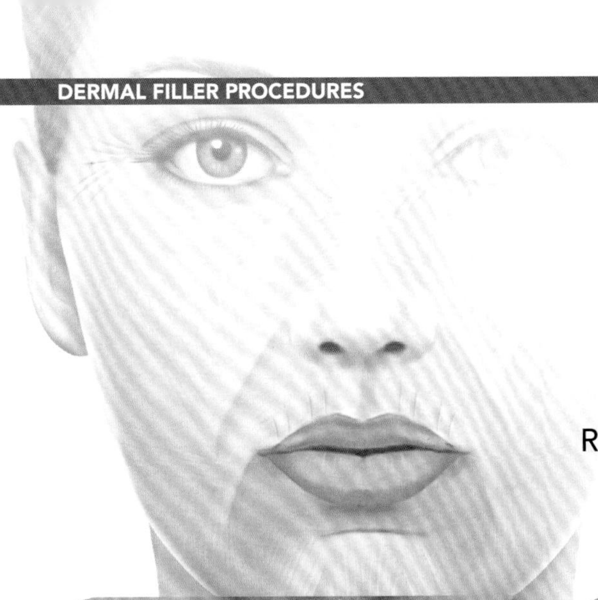

# Chapter 7

# Lip Body

### Rebecca Small, M.D.

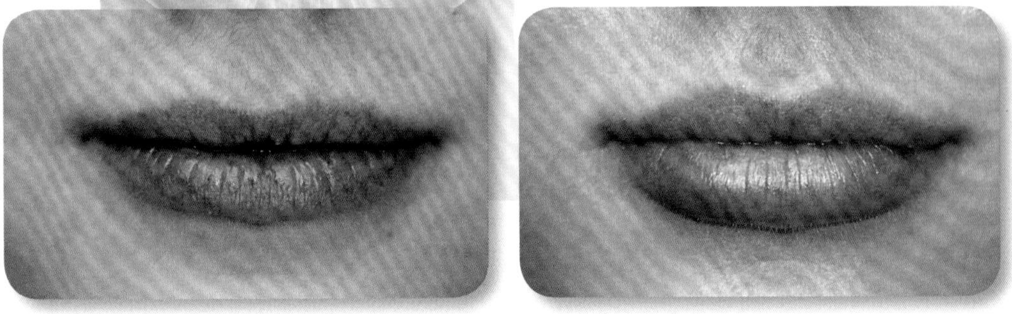

**FIGURE 1** ● Lip fullness before **(A)** and 4 weeks after **(B)** dermal filler treatment of the lip body, using hyaluronic acid.

Using proper technique and products, dermal filler treatments can enhance lip fullness in a natural way. This procedure can benefit patients with diminished lip volume from aging, as well as younger patients for enhancement purposes.

## Indications

- Lip atrophy

## Anatomy

- **Wrinkles, folds, and contours.** The pink area of the lip is called the vermillion, and is composed of dry and wet mucosa. With the mouth closed, the dry mucosa is exposed to the air and the wet mucosa remains inside the mouth. The junction between these two portions of the lip vermillion is called the wet–dry border. Lip shape and fullness varies widely. In general, the lower lip is more full than the upper lip. According to aesthetic norms, the upper lip height in the anterior-posterior view is slightly more than half the size of the lower lip.

109

## Patient Assessment

- Careful consultation and examination, using a mirror, is necessary to determine lip features that the patient would like enhanced, discuss realistic expectations and advise about aesthetic outcomes. The following points are typically included:
  - A given lip shape can only be enhanced with dermal filler treatment, it cannot be altered into another lip shape.
  - With age, volume loss is more apparent in the upper lip than the lower lip, and some patients may only require treatment of the upper lip.
  - Enhancing the lip body involves placement of dermal filler in the mucosa of the lip.
  - Defining the lip shape and the line around the lips involves dermal filler placement in the vermillion border.
  - Lip augmentation often combines enhancement of both, the lip body and the lip border (see Lip Border chapter).

## Contraindications

- See Contraindications in the Introduction and Foundation Concepts section.
- **Braces.** Braces on the teeth can distort lip projection and it is best to avoid dermal filler treatment if they are present.

## Treatment Goals

- Natural fuller appearance to the lip without excessive anterior projection or lip eversion. Lip fullness should be congruent with the patient's age.

## Recommended Dermal Filler Product

- Hyaluronic acid (HA) dermal filler products with lidocaine (HA-lidocaine) that have a soft tissue filling effect are recommended for treatment of the lip body, such as Juvederm® Ultra XC or Prevelle® Silk (see Basic and Advanced Procedures in the Introduction and Foundation Concepts section). Other HA-lidocaine products, such as Juvederm® Ultra Plus XC or Restylane-L®, may also be used, and are more suitable for younger patients (ages 20s–30s) who have greater baseline tissue density and lip volume.
- This chapter describes lip body treatment with Juvederm Ultra Plus XC (HA-lidocaine).

## Dermal Filler Treatment Volumes

- The estimated HA dermal filler volume necessary for treatment is based on patients' observed facial anatomy and volume loss in the treatment area.
- Treatment of the body of the upper and lower lips typically requires 0.5–0.8 mL Juvederm Ultra XC, Juvederm Ultra Plus XC, or Restylane-L.

## Equipment for Anesthesia

- Lip ring block supplies (see Equipment for Injectable Anesthetics in the Anesthesia section)
- Lidocaine HCl 2% with epinephrine 1:100,000 buffered or unbuffered (referred to as 2% lidocaine-epinephrine solution)
- 30-gauge, ½-inch needle

## Equipment for Dermal Filler Procedure

- General dermal filler injection supplies (see Equipment in the Introduction and Foundation Concepts section)
- 30-gauge, ½-inch needle

## Anesthesia Overview

- **Lip ring block.** Adequate anesthesia of the lip prior to dermal filler injection is essential for successful lip body treatments. Patients usually require profound lip anesthesia. Dermal fillers formulated with lidocaine do not offer sufficient pain control for lip filler treatments and a lip ring block is required (see Lip Ring Block in the Anesthesia section).

## Dermal Filler Procedure Overview

- **Overview.** An overview of injection points and injection technique for treatment of the lip body is shown in Figure 2. If treating both the lip border (see Lip Border chapter) and lip body, perform treatment of the lip border first and then treat the lip body. As lip edema can occur rapidly, it is preferable to complete both procedures on one side of lip before proceeding to the opposite side.
- **Number of injections.** There are four linear thread injections for the upper lip body, and three linear thread injections for the lower lip body—a total of seven injections (see Techniques for Dermal Filler Injection in the Introduction and Foundation Concepts section).

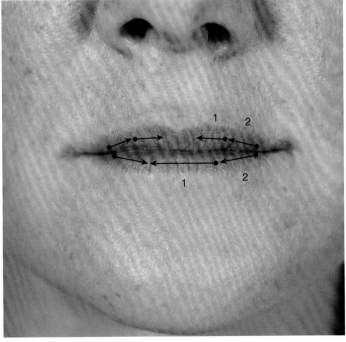

✔ = Dermal filler injection

*FIGURE 2* ● Overview of lip body dermal filler injections.

- **Depth of injection.** Dermal filler is injected 2–3 mm deep in the mucosa, at or just superior to the wet–dry border, for treatment of the lip body.
- **Cautions**
  - Observe filler volumes closely during treatment and administer equal volumes on both sides of the lips, unless gross asymmetry is present prior to treatment.
  - Lip edema can occur rapidly. At completion of the treatment, the side injected first may appear larger due to edema. If asymmetry is evident at the completion of treatment, and injection volumes and palpable product have been consistent for both sides, then it is advisable to reassess symmetry at the follow-up visit once edema has resolved.
  - Care must be taken to avoid the labial arteries, which are located deep in the labial mucosa, as intravascular dermal filler injection can result in vascular occlusion, tissue ischemia, and necrosis.

## Performing the Procedure: Dermal Filler Treatment of the Lip Body

### Anesthesia

1. Clean and prepare the lips with alcohol, removing all lipstick if present.
2. Perform a lip ring block (see Lip Ring Block in the Anesthesia section) as follows:
   - For the upper lip, use a total volume of 1.2-mL 2% lidocaine-epinephrine solution.
   - For the lower lip, use a total volume of 1.2-mL 2% lidocaine-epinephrine solution.
   - For the corners of the lips, use a total volume of 0.2-mL 2% lidocaine-epinephrine solution.
3. Wait 3–5 minutes for anesthesia.

### Dermal Filler Upper Lip Body

1. Position the patient in a 60-degree reclined position.
2. Prepare the lips with alcohol.
3. Attach a 30-gauge, ½-inch needle to the prefilled HA-lidocaine dermal filler syringe. Ensure that the needle is firmly affixed to the dermal filler syringe to prevent the needle popping off when plunger pressure is applied.
4. Prime the needle by depressing the syringe plunger until a small amount of dermal filler extrudes from the needle tip.
5. The provider is positioned on the same side as the lip area to be injected.
6. Identify the first injection point in the body of the upper lip by laying the needle against the mucosa at the wet–dry border, such that the needle tip ends at the ipsilateral peak of the Cupid's bow. The injection point is at the needle hub.
7. Insert the needle into the lip mucosa at a 30-degree angle to the lip, directing it parallel to the lip body and medially toward the ipsilateral peak of the Cupid's bow. The needle is inserted to the hub and a linear thread of filler is injected by applying firm and constant pressure on the syringe plunger while gradually withdrawing needle. The filler should flow easily into the lip mucosa and the lip will subtly fill as the product is injected (Fig. 3).
8. The second injection point in the body of the upper lip is one needle length lateral to the first injection point. The needle is inserted to the hub and the filler is smoothly injected as the needle is withdrawn (Fig. 4).

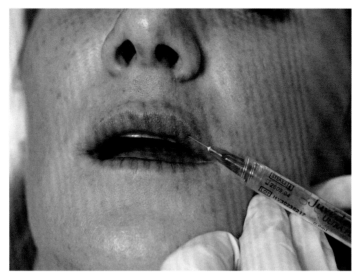

FIGURE 3 ● First injection for dermal filler treatment of the upper lip body.

9. Gently grasp the lip with thumb on the skin and first finger intraorally, and slowly compress from medial to lateral along the length of the lip to smooth any visible or palpable bumps of filler product. If bumps do not easily compress, the area may be moistened with water and stretched between the provider's fingers. Additional swelling and bruising commonly occur after compression and manipulation of filler product.

10. Reposition to the opposite side of the patient, and repeat the above injections for the contralateral upper lip body.

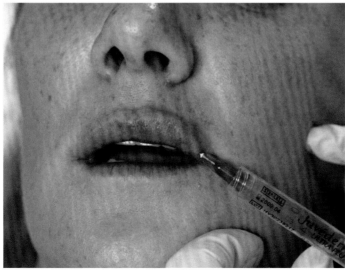

FIGURE 4 ● Second injection for dermal filler treatment of the upper lip body.

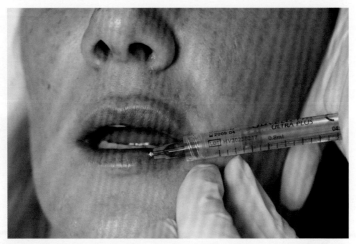

**FIGURE 5** ● First injection for dermal filler treatment of the lower lip body.

## Dermal Filler Lower Lip Body

1. Repeat steps 1–5 as listed above.
2. Identify the first injection point in the body of the lower lip by laying the needle against the mucosa at the wet–dry border such that the length of the needle spans the center portion of the lower lip. The injection point is at the needle's hub.
3. Insert the needle into the lip mucosa at a 30-degree angle to the lip, and direct it parallel to the lip and medially across the center portion of the lower lip body. The needle is inserted to the hub and the filler is smoothly injected as the needle is withdrawn (Fig. 5).
4. The second injection point in the body of the lower lip is one needle length lateral to the first injection point. The needle is inserted to the hub and the filler is smoothly injected as the needle is withdrawn (Fig. 6).

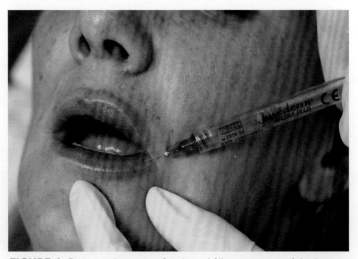

**FIGURE 6** ● Second injection for dermal filler treatment of the lower lip body.

5. Reposition to the opposite side of the patient, and repeat the above injections for the contralateral lower lip body.
6. Gently compress the lip from medial to lateral as described above.

## Tip

- Watch for tissue blanching or other ischemic signs or symptoms with injection of the lips. If ischemia occurs, manage as described in Complications, Tissue Ischemia section.

## Results

- Lip augmentation is evident at the time of treatment. Immediately after injection, lips may appear overfilled and project anteriorly due to edema. Once edema resolves, lips will appear more full than at baseline, and will be anatomically positioned (see Lip Border section, Fig. 1A, B and C).

## Duration of Effects and Subsequent Treatments

- Lip augmentation typically lasts 6–9 months after treatment, as this is a highly mobile region.
- Subsequent treatment with dermal filler is recommended when the volume of dermal filler product is visibly diminished.

## Follow-ups and Management

Patients are assessed 4 weeks after treatment to evaluate for adequacy of lip augmentation and symmetry. Common issues reported by patients include the following:

- **Bruising, swelling, erythema, and tenderness.** See Follow-ups and Management in Introduction and Foundation Concepts section. Lip edema typically resolves within 3–5 days. Patients often require reassurance to this effect. Application of ice immediately after the procedure and as directed in the aftercare instructions (Appendix 2) can reduce swelling.
- **Mild lip asymmetry.** Asymmetry may be due to too little or too much filler in some areas.
  - **Additional filler required.** Identify the areas where more filler is desired, both visually and by palpation. The small region requiring a touch up can be anesthetized using the lip ring block method by placing lidocaine intraorally adjacent to the region where the touch up is required. The amount necessary for the touch up will vary based on the volume deficit, and it is typically 0.1–0.3 mL of HA-lidocaine.
  - **Too much filler or uneven placement.** Small collections of filler can usually be compressed and smoothed. Large collections may require hyaluronidase injection or, as a last resort, incision and expression of product (see Complications section).

## Complications and Management

- General dermal filler complications and management are reviewed the Complications section
- Swelling and bruising

- Oral herpes simplex reactivation
- Tissue ischemia and necrosis

**Significant swelling and bruising** are the most common side effects with lip augmentation dermal filler treatments (see Complications section, and Follow-ups and Management in the Introduction and Foundation Concepts section).

**Reactivation of oral herpes simplex** is not uncommon and prophylactic antiviral therapy typically suppresses reactivation (see Preprocedure Checklist in the Introduction and Foundation Concepts section).

**Tissue ischemia and necrosis** can result from intravascular dermal filler injection of the labial arteries. With age and associated loss of lip volume, these vessels lie closer to the labial mucosa and the risk of intravascular injection increases (see Complications section).

## Combining Aesthetic Treatments and Maximizing Results

- **Botulinum toxin.** The orbicularis oris muscle which encircles the mouth, functions to pucker lips and invert the vermillion border, and over time, repetitive contraction can contribute to reduced lip volume radial lip line formation. Botulinum toxin treatment of the orbicularis oris muscle is commonly used adjunctively with dermal fillers for lip augmentation, as it everts lips slightly and enhances lip fullness.
- **Dermal filler in adjacent areas.** Enhanced lip fullness can be achieved with concurrent dermal filler treatment of the lip body and lip border (see Lip Border chapter).

## Pricing

Dermal filler fees are based on the type of filler used, size and number of syringes, injector's skill, and vary according to community pricing in different geographic regions. Prices range from $500 to $800 per syringe of 0.8 mL HA for lip augmentation treatment.

# Chapter 8

# Lip Lines

### Rebecca Small, M.D.

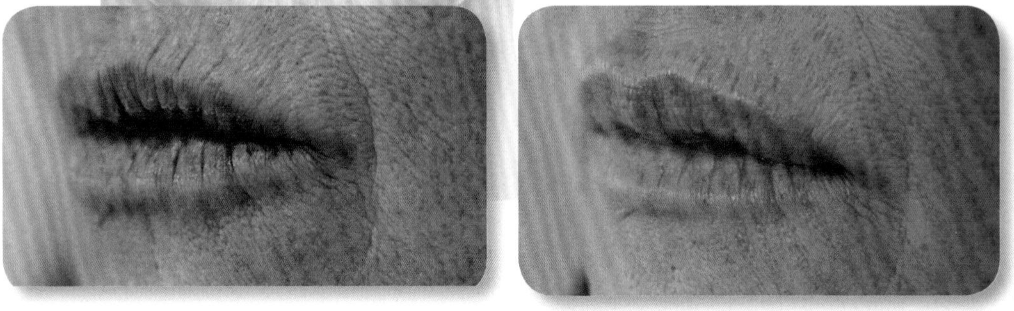

A       B

*FIGURE 1* ● Lip lines before **(A)** and 4 weeks after **(B)** dermal filler treatment, using calcium hydroxylapatite above the lip and hyaluronic acid in the lip vermillion border.

Perioral lip lines, particularly in the upper lip, are commonly seen with aging. Using proper technique and products, dermal filler treatments can reduce perioral lip lines resulting in a smooth natural appearance. Although lip lines can form on both the upper and lower lips, upper lip lines are most problematic for patients, and this chapter, therefore, focuses on treatment of the upper lip region. Two types of filler products are used with the technique described in this chapter. A dermal filler with more structural support is placed above the upper lip, and a more supple dermal filler product is placed in the lip border. These more complex techniques are considered advanced dermal filler procedures.

## Indications

- Perioral rhytids

## Anatomy

- **Wrinkles, folds, and contours.** Lip lines, or perioral rhytids, form perpendicular to the lip and radiate away from the vermillion border (see Dermal Filler Anatomy section, Figs. 1 and 2). Many factors contribute to formation of lip lines including: perioral soft tissue volume loss, lip atrophy, hyperdynamic perioral musculature, and biometric volume loss due to resorption of mandibular bone and tooth alveolar processes.

**117**

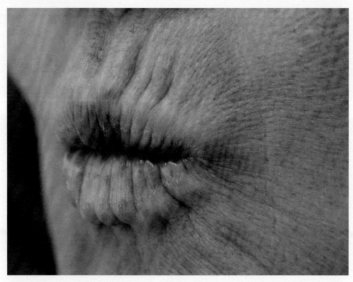

FIGURE 2 ● Dynamic lip lines.

## Patient Assessment

- Careful consultation and examination using a mirror is necessary to assess lip and peri-oral aging changes, discuss realistic expectations and advise about aesthetic outcomes.
- Patients with static lines typically have significant hyperdynamic perioral musculature as well as volume loss (Fig. 2). Optimal reduction of lip lines usually consists of treatment with botulinum toxin and dermal filler (see Combining Aesthetic Treatments and Maximizing Results below).
- Patients with very thin, diminutive upper lips often benefit from dermal filler treatment above the lip only. Treatment of the lip border in these patients can result in an unnatural anterior projection of the upper lip or a "duck" lip.

## Contraindications

- See Contraindications in the Introduction and Foundation Concepts section.
- **Braces.** Braces on the teeth can distort lip projection and it is best to avoid dermal filler treatment if they are present.

## Treatment Goals

- Natural lip appearance with reduction of lip lines and defined lip border without excessive anterior projection or lip eversion.

## Recommended Dermal Filler Product

- The region above the upper lip is ideally treated with dermal filler products that offer significant structural support such as Radiesse®, which is a calcium hydroxylapatite (CaHA) product. Products that provide moderate structural support, such as Juvederm® Ultra Plus and Restylane®, which are hyaluronic acid (HA) products, can also be used (see Basic and Advanced Procedures in the Introduction and Foundation Concepts section).

- Filling the lip border can be achieved using a dermal filler product that has a softer tissue fill such as Juvederm® Ultra XC or Prevelle® Silk (hyaluronic acid-lidocaine). Patients requiring treatment of lip lines typically have lip atrophy and the firmer HA products are less appropriate (see Products and Basic and Advanced Procedures in the Introduction and Foundation Concepts section).
- This chapter describes treatment of upper lip lines with the following products:
  - **Above the upper lip** is treated with Radiesse (CaHA), in particular CaHA that has been mixed with a small amount of lidocaine (CaHA-lidocaine)
  - **Upper lip border** is treated with Juvederm Ultra XC (HA-lidocaine).

## Dermal Filler Treatment Volumes

- The estimated dermal filler volume necessary for treatment is based on patients' observed facial anatomy and volume loss in the treatment area.
- Treatment above the upper lip typically requires 0.3–0.4 mL CaHA-lidocaine (Radiesse®).
- Treatment of the medial vermillion border of the upper lip typically requires 0.3–0.4 mL HA-lidocaine (Juvederm® Ultra XC).

## Equipment for Anesthesia

- Lip Ring Block supplies (see Equipment for Injectable Anesthetics in the Anesthesia section)
- Lidocaine HCl 2% with epinephrine 1:100,000 buffered or unbuffered (referred to as 2% lidocaine-epinephrine solution)
- 30-gauge, ½-inch needle

## Equipment for Dermal Filler Procedure

- General dermal filler injection supplies (see Equipment in the Introduction and Foundation Concepts section)
- CaHA mixing supplies (see Equipment in the Introduction and Foundation Concepts section)
- 27-gauge, 1½-inch needle
- 30-gauge, ½-inch needle

## Anesthesia Overview

- **Lip ring block.** Adequate anesthesia of the lip prior to dermal filler injection is essential for successful lip line treatments. Patients usually require profound lip anesthesia. Dermal fillers formulated or mixed with lidocaine do not offer sufficient pain control for lip filler treatments and a lip ring block is required (see Lip Ring Block in the Anesthesia section).

## Dermal Filler Procedure Overview

- **Overview.** An overview of injection points and injection technique for treatment of upper lip lines is shown in Figure 3. Treatment of lip lines is achieved with dermal filler injection above the upper lip and into the lip vermillion border. This method reduces the appearance of lip lines by volumizing the upper lip area.
- **CaHA-lidocaine preparation** is performed at the time of treatment (see Calcium Hydroxylapatite and Lidocaine Preparation in the in Introduction and Foundation Concepts section)

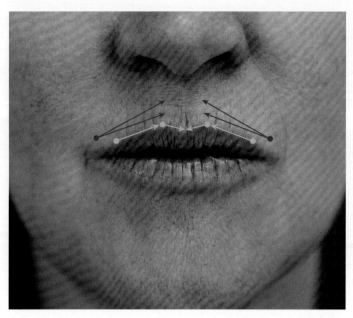

= Calcium hydroxylapatite dermal filler        = Hyaluronic acid dermal filler

*FIGURE 3* ● Overview of lip line dermal filler injections.

- **Number of injections and injection depth.**
  - **Above the upper lip** is treated with two fanning injections using CaHA-lidocaine. Injections are placed in the mid- to deep dermis.
  - **The vermillion border** is treated with four linear thread injections using HA-lidocaine (see Techniques for Dermal Filler Injection in the Introduction and Foundation Concepts section). Injections are placed in the superficial dermis of the vermillion border.
- **Cautions**
  - Observe filler volumes closely during treatment and administer equal volumes on both sides of the lips, unless gross asymmetry is present prior to treating.
  - Care should be taken to avoid injection into the vermillion border or the lip mucosa with CaHA, as there are reports of nodules with Radiesse injected in the lip.
  - Perioral and lip edema can occur rapidly. If significant edema is evident after placing CaHA-lidocaine above the upper lip, discontinue further treatment and assess lip lines at the follow-up visit in 2–4 weeks. In addition, the side injected first may appear larger at the completion of treatment due to edema. If asymmetry is evident at the completion of treatment, and injections volumes and palpable product have been consistent for both sides, then it is advisable to reassess symmetry at the follow-up visit once edema has resolved.

## Performing the Procedure: Dermal Filler Treatment of Lip Lines

### Anesthesia

1. Clean and prepare the lips with alcohol, removing all lipstick if present.
2. Perform a lip ring block (see Lip Ring Block in the Anesthesia section) as follows:

- For the upper lip, use a total volume of 1.2-mL 2% lidocaine-epinephrine solution.
- For the lower lip, use a total volume of 1.2-mL 2% lidocaine-epinephrine solution.
- For the corners of the lips, use a total volume of 0.2-mL 2% lidocaine-epinephrine solution.

3. Wait 3–5 minutes for anesthesia.

## Dermal Filler Above the Upper Lip

1. Position the patient in a 60-degree reclined position.
2. Prepare the lips with alcohol.
3. The provider is positioned on the same side as the lip to be injected.
4. Use a prepared CaHA-lidocaine dermal filler syringe and attach a 27-gauge, 1½-inch needle to the syringe. Ensure that the needle is firmly affixed to the dermal filler syringe to prevent the needle popping off when plunger pressure is applied.
5. Prime the needle by depressing the syringe plunger until a small amount of dermal filler extrudes from the needle tip.
6. Identify the first injection point above the lip by laying the needle 3–4 mm superior and parallel to the vermillion border, such that the needle tip ends at the ipsilateral peak of the Cupid's bow. The first injection point is at the needle hub (Fig. 4A).
7. Insert the needle at a 30-degree angle to the skin and direct it medially toward the peak of the ipsilateral Cupid's bow and parallel to the lip (Fig. 4B). Apply firm and constant pressure on the syringe plunger while gradually withdrawing needle to inject a linear thread of filler in the mid- to deep dermis. Fan the needle superiorly without fully withdrawing the needle from the skin to inject another linear thread, using small angulations to ensure that dermal filler placement is contiguous.
8. Gently grasp the lip with the thumb on the skin and first finger intraorally, and slowly compress from medial to lateral along the length of the lip, to smooth any visible or palpable bumps of filler product. If bumps do not easily compress, the area may be moistened with water and stretched between the provider's fingers. Additional swelling and bruising commonly occur after compression and manipulation of filler product in the lip area.
9. Reposition to the opposite side and repeat the above injections for contralateral area above the upper lip.

## Dermal Filler Lip Border

1. The provider is positioned on the same side to be injected.
2. Use a prefilled HA-lidocaine syringe and attach a 30-gauge, ½-inch needle.
3. Identify the first lip border injection point by laying the needle against the vermillion border such that the needle tip ends at the ipsilateral peak of the Cupid's bow. The needle insertion point is at the needle hub. Insert the needle into the vermillion border at a 30-degree angle to the lip and direct it toward the ipsilateral peak of the Cupid's bow (Fig. 5). Apply firm and constant pressure on the syringe plunger while gradually withdrawing needle to inject a linear thread of filler. The filler should flow easily into the vermillion border and a rolled border to the lip will be visible as the filler product is injected. Figure 6 shows the left vermillion border immediately after treatment.
4. The second lip border injection point is at the ipsilateral peak of the Cupid's bow. Insert the needle and advance inferior-medially to the nadir of the Cupid's bow. Smoothly inject a small amount of filler as the needle is withdrawn.

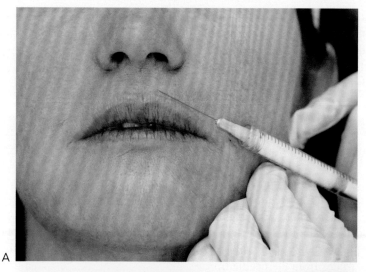

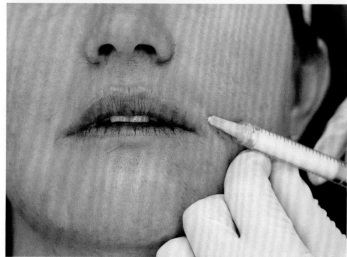

*FIGURE 4* ● Injection above the upper lip for dermal filler treatment of
lip lines: needle insertion point determination **(A)** and injection technique **(B).**

5. Gently grasp the lip with thumb on the skin and first finger intraorally, and slowly
   compress from medial to lateral along the length of the lip to smooth any visible
   or palpable bumps of filler product. If bumps do not easily compress, the area may
   be moistened with water and stretched between the provider's fingers. Additional
   swelling and bruising commonly occur after compression and manipulation of filler
   product.
6. Reposition to the opposite side and repeat the above injections for the contralateral
   upper lip border.

## Tips

- Filler should be smooth and confluent in the vermillion border. If there is a visible or
  palpable skipped area, inject this area using the earlier technique until filler product
  is contiguous and desired correction is achieved.

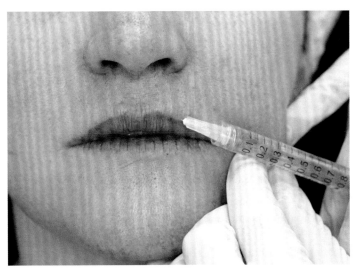

*FIGURE 5* ● Injection in the lip border for dermal filler treatment of lip lines.

## Results

- Reduction of lip lines is evident at the time of treatment. However, immediately after injection, the upper lip may appear overfilled and project anteriorly due to edema. Once edema resolves, lips will appear more defined with reduced radial lip lines. Figure 1 shows a 46-year-old woman with lip lines before (A) and 4 weeks after (B) treatment with 0.3 mL CaHA-lidocaine (Radiesse) above the upper lip and 0.3 mL HA-lidocaine (Juvederm Ultra XC) in the vermillion border of the upper lip.

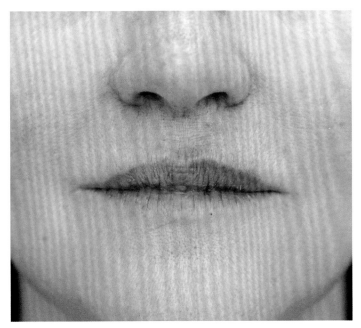

*FIGURE 6* ● Left upper lip border immediately after dermal filler treatment with hyaluronic acid.

## Duration of Effects and Subsequent Treatments

- Reduction of lip lines with dermal filler typically lasts 9–12 months after treatment, as this is a highly mobile region.
- Subsequent treatment with dermal filler is recommended when the volume of dermal filler product is visibly diminished, prior to their pretreatment appearance.

## Follow-ups and Management

Patients are assessed 4 weeks after treatment to evaluate for adequacy of lip augmentation and symmetry. Common issues reported by patients include the following:

- **Bruising, swelling, erythema, and tenderness.** See Follow-ups and Management in the Introduction and Foundation Concepts section. Lip edema typically resolves within 3–5 days. Patients often require reassurance to this effect. Application of ice immediately after the procedure and as directed in the aftercare instructions (Appendix 2) can reduce swelling.
- **Mild lip asymmetry.** Asymmetry may be due to too little or too much filler in some areas.
  - **Additional filler required.** Identify the areas where more filler is desired, both visually and by palpation. The small region requiring a touch-up can be anesthetized using the lip ring block method by placing lidocaine intraorally adjacent to the region where the touch-up is required. The amount necessary for the touch-up will vary based on the volume deficit, and it is typically 0.1–0.2 mL CaHA-lidocaine or 0.1–0.2 mL HA-lidocaine.
  - **Too much filler or uneven placement.** Small collections of filler can usually be compressed and smoothed. Large collections of HA may require hyaluronidase injection, or as a last resort, HA and CaHA collections may be incised and product expressed (see Complications section).

## Complications and Management

- General dermal filler complications and management are reviewed in the Complications section
- Swelling and bruising
- Oral herpes simplex reactivation

   **Significant swelling and bruising** are the most common side effects with lip augmentation dermal filler treatments (see Complications section, and Follow-ups and Management in the Introduction and Foundation Concepts section).

   **Reactivation of oral herpes simplex** is not uncommon and prophylactic antiviral therapy typically suppresses reactivation (see Preprocedure Checklist in the Introduction and Foundation Concepts section).

## Combining Aesthetic Treatments and Maximizing Results

- **Botulinum toxin.** The orbicularis oris muscle, which encircles the mouth functions to pucker lips, can contribute to lip line formation. Botulinum toxin treatment of the orbicularis oris muscle is commonly performed adjunctively to reduce lip lines and enhance lip fullness as it everts lips slightly.

- **Skin resurfacing and collagen stimulating treatments.** Reduction of lip lines can often be improved by combining dermal fillers with skin resurfacing or collagen stimulating procedures such as ablative and nonablative lasers, dermabrasion, and chemical peels. With the more aggressive procedures such as ablative and fractional ablative lasers, dermabrasion, and medium depth chemical peels, dermal filler treatments are performed after recovery. With less aggressive procedures such as nonablative lasers, superficial chemical peels, and microdermabrasion, dermal filler treatments may be performed in the same visit or prior to these procedures.

## Pricing

Dermal filler fees are based on the type of filler used, size and number of syringes, injector's skill, and vary according to community pricing in different geographic regions. Prices range from $500 to $800 per syringe of 0.8 mL HA and $650 to $850 per syringe of 0.8 mL CaHA for lip line treatment.

# Chapter 9

# Malar Augmentation

Rebecca Small, M.D.

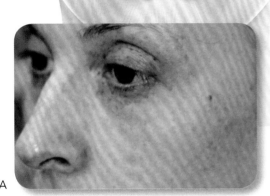
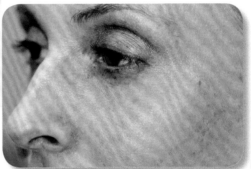

A

B

FIGURE 1 ● Malar region before **(A)** and 4 weeks after **(B)** dermal filler malar augmentation, using calcium hydroxylapatite.

A flat malar area can make the face appear tired and sunken, and contribute to a prematurely aged appearance. Treatment of a flat malar area has traditionally been a surgical procedure utilizing malar implants. Dermal fillers can also be used to successfully restore midface fullness and enhance malar contours. Malar augmentation utilizes dermal filler products that offer more structural support, and is considered an advanced dermal filler procedure.

## Indications

• Malar atrophy and flattening

## Anatomy

• **Wrinkles, folds, and contour changes.** Over time, the convex contour of the midface region can flatten or become concave (see Dermal Filler Anatomy section, Figs. 1 and 2). Descent of the malar soft tissue complex from the zygoma and orbital rims inferomedially, and malar fat pad atrophy contribute to these contour changes. The malar groove (Figs. 3A and 3B), also called the zygomatic hollow, is a linear depression that runs diagonally across the zygoma, parallel to the nasolabial fold. It corresponds to a deep ligament attachment (zygomaticomalar ligament) and can become more apparent over time with midface tissue atrophy

127

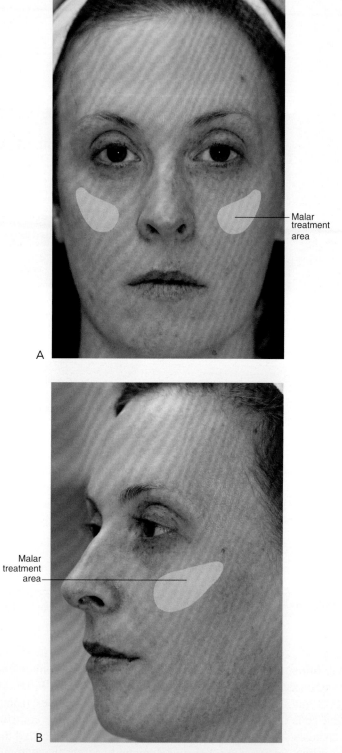

A

Malar
treatment
area

Malar
treatment
area

B

*FIGURE 2* ● Malar augmentation treatment area from the front **(A)**
and lateral **(B)** views.

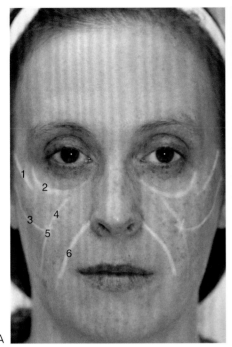
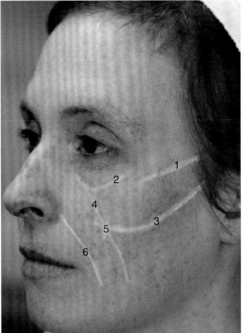

A

B

1. Superior zygoma margin      4. Malar groove
2. Orbital rim                 5. First injection point
3. Inferior zygoma margin      6. Nasolabial fold

**FIGURE 3** ● Facial landmarks for dermal filler malar augmentation from the front **(A)** and lateral **(B)** views.

and descent. The infraorbital vein, artery, and nerve are located along the midpupillary line approximately 2.5 cm below the inferior orbital rim (see Dermal Filler Anatomy section, Figs. 3 and 4).

# Patient Assessment

- Malar contour is assessed from the anterior (Fig. 2A) and 45-degree views (Fig. 2B). A desirable malar contour is convex and not flat.

# Contraindications

- See Contraindications in Introduction and Foundation Concepts section.

## Treatment Goals

- Increased anterior projection and convexity of the malar region.

# Recommended Dermal Filler Product

- This is an area of deep volume loss and is ideally treated with advanced dermal filler products that offer more structural support such as Radiesse® (calcium hydroxylapatite [CaHA]) or Perlane-L® (hyaluronic acid [HA]) (see Basic and Advanced Procedures in the Introduction and Foundation Concepts section).

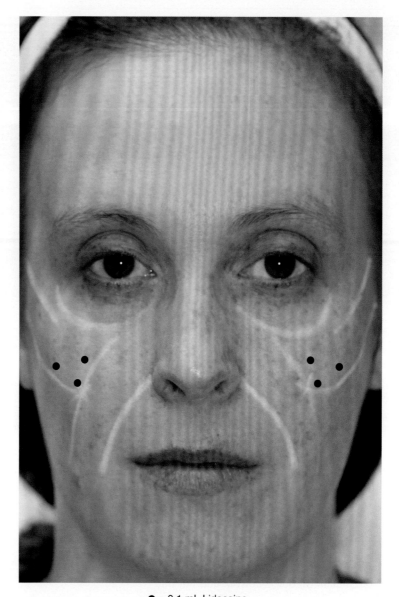

● = 0.1 mL Lidocaine

*FIGURE 4* ● Anesthesia for malar augmentation dermal filler treatment.

- This chapter describes malar augmentation with CaHA (Radiesse), in particular CaHA that has been mixed with a small amount of lidocaine (CaHA-lidocaine). CaHA-lidocaine has reduced viscosity and a mild anesthetic effect (see Calcium Hydroxylapatite and Lidocaine Preparation in the Introduction and Foundation Concepts section).

## Dermal Filler Treatment Volumes

- The estimated CaHA-lidocaine (Radiesse) dermal filler volume necessary for treatment is based on the patient's observed facial anatomy and volume loss in the treatment area.
- Malar augmentation typically requires 2.0–2.6 mL CaHA-lidocaine.

## Equipment for Anesthesia

- Local infiltration injection supplies (see Equipment for Injectable Anesthetics in the Anesthesia section)
- Lidocaine HCl 2% with epinephrine 1:100,000 buffered (referred to as buffered 2% lidocaine-epinephrine solution)
- 30-gauge, ½-inch needle

## Equipment for Dermal Filler Procedure

- General dermal filler injection supplies (see Equipment in the Introduction and Foundation Concepts section)
- CaHA (Radiesse) with lidocaine mixing supplies (see Equipment in the Introduction and Foundation Concepts section)
- 28-gauge, ¾-inch needle

## Landmarks

Facial landmarks are marked on the patient at rest using a soft white eyeliner pencil including the nasolabial folds, malar grooves which run parallel to the nasolabial folds, inferior orbital rims, and margins of the zygoma (Figs. 3A and 3B). Note that the zygoma is oriented horizontally in the midface and angulates superior laterally towards the ear. All injections are placed along the zygoma bone. Palpate the inferior margin zygoma in the midface and follow it superolaterally to create a mental map of the bone.

## Anesthesia Overview

- **Local lidocaine infiltration.** Buffered 2% lidocaine-epinephrine solution can be used to achieve anesthesia for malar augmentation. The malar area is anesthetized using six injections of 0.1 mL for a total volume of 0.6 mL (Fig. 4). See Injectable Anesthetics in the Anesthesia section for additional information on local infiltration methods.

## Overview of Dermal Filler Procedure

- **Overview.** Malar augmentation targets the flattened cheek area and malar groove (Figs. 2A and 2B). An overview of malar augmentation injection points and injection technique is shown in Figures 5A and B.
- **Number of injections.** There are five depot injections on each side of the face (see Techniques for Dermal Filler Injection in the Introduction and Foundation Concepts section). The five injections are distributed in two rows that form a roughly triangular region, with the base located approximately 2 cm lateral to the nasolabial fold, and the tip superolateral along the zygoma.
- **Injection depth and volume.** Dermal filler is placed in the supraperiosteal plane for malar augmentation using the depot injection technique. The needle is inserted through the skin and muscle, and advanced until a gentle tap is felt against the bone. The needle is then withdrawn 1–2 mm, and a bolus of product is placed just above the bone. The volume placed at each injection point is determined by the depth of the

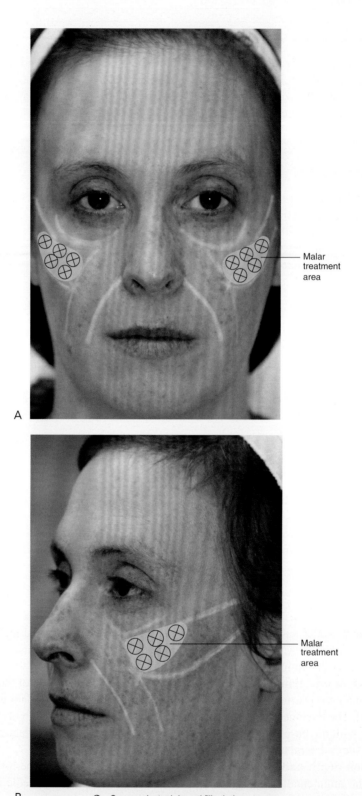

Malar
treatment
area

A

Malar
treatment
area

B                ⊕ = Supraperiosteal dermal filler bolus

*FIGURE 5* ● Overview of dermal filler injections for malar augmentation seen from the front **(A)** and lateral **(B)** views.

28-gauge, ¾-inch needle in tissue. Deeper injection points receive greater volumes. The medial injection points are usually deeper than the lateral sites.

- **Cautions**
  - The region between the ala and nasolabial fold is avoided with malar augmentation, as dermal filler in this area can accentuate the nasolabial fold.
  - The infraorbital vein, artery, and nerve are avoided with malar augmentation.

## Performing the Procedure: Dermal Filler Malar Augmentation

### Anesthesia

1. Clean and prepare the skin in the extended mental crease area with alcohol.
2. Inject buffered 2% lidocaine-epinephrine solution subcutaneously as shown in Figure 4.
3. Allow a few minutes for anesthesia.

### Dermal Filler

1. Position the patient in a 45-degree reclined position.
2. Clean and prepare the skin of the malar region with alcohol.
3. The provider is positioned on the same side as the malar area to be injected.
4. Attach a 28-gauge, ¾-inch needle to the CaHA-lidocaine dermal filler syringe. Ensure that the needle is firmly affixed to the dermal filler syringe to prevent the needle popping off when plunger pressure is applied.
5. Prime the needle by depressing the syringe plunger until a small amount of dermal filler extrudes from the needle tip.
6. The first injection point is at the intersection of the malar groove line and the inferior margin of the zygoma. Insert the needle at 45 degrees to the skin and direct it posteriorly toward the zygoma bone. Advance to the needle until bone is felt as a soft tap. Withdraw the needle 1–2 mm and, using the depot technique, inject with firm and constant pressure on the syringe plunger (Fig. 6). If the needle is inserted to:
   - Full depth, inject 0.2–0.3 mL CaHA-lidocaine
   - Half depth or less, inject 0.1 mL CaHA-lidocaine.
     After depositing the desired volume of product, discontinue injection and then remove the needle.
7. The second injection point is approximately 1 cm superolateral to the first, along the inferior zygoma. Inject as described above.
8. The third injection point, which is the last injection in this row, is approximately 1 cm superolateral to the second, along the inferior zygoma. Inject as above.
9. The fourth injection point begins the superior row of injections and is approximately 1 cm superior and slightly medial to the first injection point. Inject as above.
10. The fifth injection point is approximately 1 cm superolateral to the fourth injection point. Inject as above.
11. Palpate the treatment area to determine whether there are any skipped areas where filler is not palpable. Inject these areas with small boluses, using the above technique, until filler product placement is contiguous and desired correction is achieved.

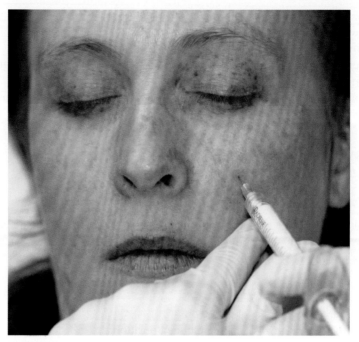

*FIGURE 6* ● Depot injection technique for malar augmentation dermal filler treatment.

12. Compress the treatment area with both thumbs on the skin using firm pressure from medial to lateral, to ensure a smooth contour to the cheek.
13. Reposition to the opposite side of the patient and repeat the above injections for the contralateral malar region.

## Tip

- Take care not to inject filler product while the needle is withdrawn as this may track product in the dermis. If the product is tracked in the dermis, squeeze the skin and express the product from the insertion site.

## Results

- Malar augmentation is immediately evident at the time of treatment. Malar augmentation results are shown in Figure 1 for a 36-year-old patient before (A) and 4 weeks after (C) treatment with 2.0-mL CaHA-lidocaine dermal filler, Radiesse.

## Duration of Effects and Subsequent Treatments

- Malar augmentation with CaHA typically lasts 1–1½ years.
- Subsequent treatment with dermal filler is recommended when the volume of filler product is visibly diminished and the malar contour begins to flatten, or the malar groove is more obvious, prior to the pretreatment appearance.

## Follow-ups and Management

Patients are assessed 4 weeks after treatment to evaluate for adequacy of malar augmentation. Common issues reported by patients include the following:

- **Bruising, swelling, erythema, and tenderness.** See Follow-up section in the Introduction and Foundation Concepts section for recommendations and management strategies.
- **Asymmetry.** Additional dermal filler may be necessary if a volume deficit is visible. A typical touch-up procedure requires 0.3–0.4 mL CaHA-lidocaine to address volume deficits. If possible, use ice or topical anesthetic for the touch-up procedure to reduce tissue distortion that can occur with local lidocaine infiltration.

## Complications and Management

- General dermal filler complications and management are reviewed the Complications section.

## Combining Aesthetic Treatments and Maximizing Results

- **Dermal filler in adjacent areas.** Patients requiring malar augmentation may also have prominent nasolabial folds. It is advisable to perform malar augmentation first and reassess nasolabial folds at the follow-up visit. Restoring midface volume can reduce nasolabial folds and hence, smaller treatment volumes for nasolabial fold correction can often be used after malar augmentation is performed (see Nasolabial Fold chapter).

## Pricing

Dermal filler fees are based on the type of filler used, size and number of syringes, the injector's skill, and vary according to community pricing in different geographic regions. Prices range from $650 to $1200 per syringe of 1.5 mL CaHA for malar augmentation.

# Chapter 10

# Frown Lines

Rebecca Small, M.D.

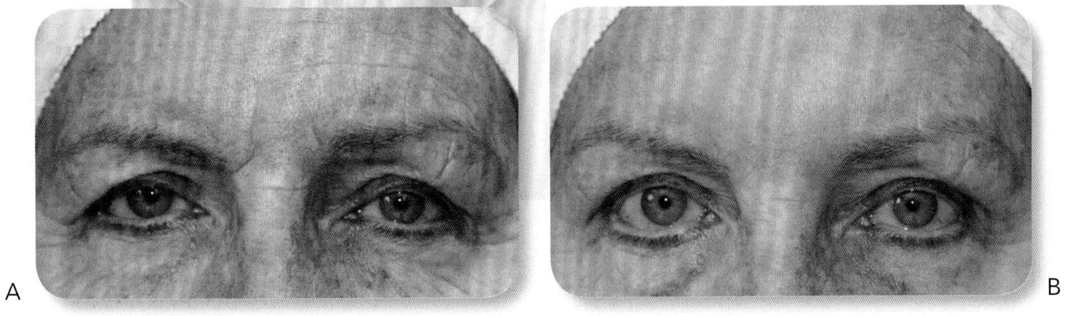

*FIGURE 1* ● Frown lines before **(A)** and 2 weeks after **(B)** dermal filler treatment using hyaluronic acid.

Frown lines convey irritation, anger, and frustration and are a common presenting complaint of patients seeking aesthetic treatments. Botulinum toxin is the treatment of choice for frown lines resulting from hyperdynamic musculature. However, static frown lines that are etched into the skin and visible at rest, respond well to dermal filler treatments.

## Indications

• Static frown lines

## Anatomy

• **Wrinkles, folds, and contours.** Frown lines, or glabellar rhytids, are vertical lines between the medial eyebrows (see Dermal Filler Anatomy section, Figs. 1 and 2). Lines and wrinkles seen only during active facial expression such as frowning, laughing, or smiling, are referred to as dynamic lines (Fig. 2A). Over time, dynamic lines can become permanently etched into skin, resulting in lines that are present at rest, which are referred to as static lines (Fig. 3B).

## Patient Assessment

• Frown lines are assessed with contraction of frown muscles and at rest to determine the dynamic and static components. Patients with predominantly dynamic frown lines

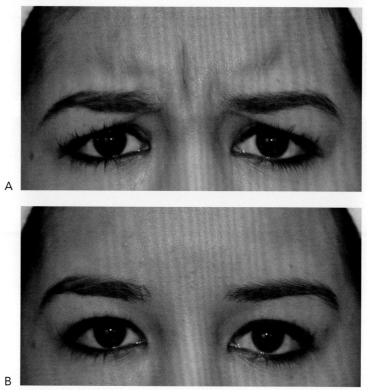

**FIGURE 2** ● Younger patient demonstrating dynamic frown lines seen with glabellar complex muscle contraction **(A)** and lack of static lines at rest **(B)** who is a poor candidate for dermal filler treatment of frown lines.

are more appropriate candidates for botulinum toxin treatment (Fig. 2). Patients with static lines usually have significant hyperdynamic musculature as well as volume loss (Fig. 3), and optimal results can be achieved with combination therapy using botulinum toxin and dermal filler (see Combining Aesthetic Treatments and Maximizing Results later).

## Contraindications

- See Contraindications in Introduction and Foundation Concepts section.

## Treatment Goals

- Reduction of static frown lines with full effacement.

## Recommended Dermal Filler Product

- Because of the risk of developing ischemia and vascular occlusion in the glabella, frown lines are best treated with the thinnest dermal fillers such as Juvederm® Ultra XC or Prevelle® Silk (see Basic and Advanced Procedures in the Introduction and Foundation Concepts section). Juvederm Ultra XC (hyaluronic acid) has a greater

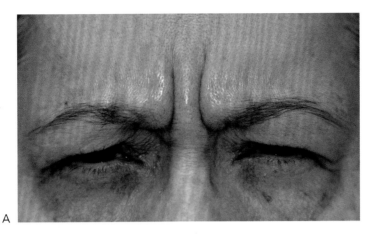

A

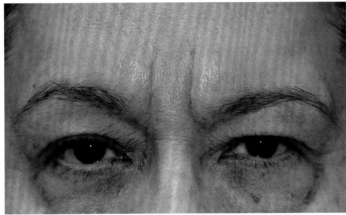

B

**FIGURE 3** ● Mother of patient in Figure 2 demonstrating dynamic frown lines seen with glabellar complex muscle contraction **(A)**, and prominent static lines at rest **(B)** who is a good candidate for dermal filler treatment of frown lines.

longevity and is currently the preferred product by the author for the treatment of frown lines.

- This chapter describes treatment of static frown lines with Juvederm Ultra XC (HA-lidocaine).

## Dermal Filler Treatment Volumes

- The estimated HA-lidocaine dermal filler volume necessary for treatment is based on patient's observed facial anatomy and volume loss in the treatment area. Small volumes are typically required for treatment of frown lines, which range from 0.2 to 0.3 mL HA-lidocaine.

## Equipment for Anesthesia

- General topical anesthetic supplies (see Equipment for Topical Anesthetics in the Anesthesia section)
- Benzocaine:lidocaine:tetracaine (BLT) ointment

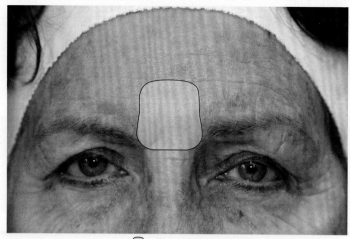

= Topical anesthetic

FIGURE 4 ● Anesthesia for frown line dermal filler treatment.

## Equipment for Dermal Filler Procedure

- General dermal filler injection supplies (see Equipment in the Introduction and Foundation Concepts section)
- 30-gauge, ½-inch needle

## Anesthesia Overview

- **Topical anesthetic.** BLT may be used to achieve anesthesia in the frown area (see Topical Anesthetics in the Anesthesia section) as shown in Figure 4.
- **Ice.** Ice is commonly used as an alternative to BLT in the frown line area.

## Dermal Filler Procedure Overview

- **Overview.** An overview of injection points and injection technique for treatment of frown lines, using a HA dermal filler, is shown in Figure 5.
- **Number of injections.** Injections are placed using the linear thread technique (see Techniques for Dermal Filler Injection in the Introduction and Foundation Concepts section). For each frown line, start with one injection at the superior most portion. If the frown line is longer than the needle length, proceed inferiorly with one additional injections. The number of injections varies according to the length of the individual patient's frown lines.
- **Injection depth.** Dermal filler is injected in the mid-dermis for treatment of frown lines.
- **Cautions.** The glabellar region is a higher risk area for ischemia and necrosis due to overfilling of tissue or vascular occlusion. Using thin dermal filler products, intradermal placement, low filler volumes, gentle plunger pressure, and keeping the needle slowly moving at all times in a retrograde fashion while injecting, may reduce the likelihood of vascular compromise in the glabellar region.

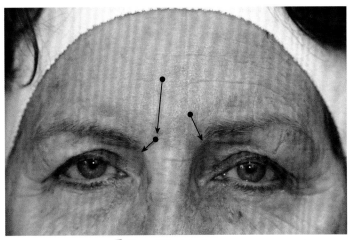

= Dermal filler injection

**FIGURE 5** ● Overview of frown line dermal filler injections.

## Performing the Procedure: Dermal Filler Treatment of Frown Lines

### Anesthesia

1. Clean and prepare the skin of the frown line area with alcohol.
2. Apply 0.5 g BLT as a thin layer to the frown area, using a cotton-tipped applicator or gloved finger (Fig. 4). Gently rub BLT, using small circular motions, to enhance penetration into the skin. Occlusion with plastic wrap is not necessary.
3. Remove BLT, 15–30 minutes after application using alcohol.

### Dermal Filler

1. Position the patient in a 45-degree reclined position.
2. Prepare the frown lines with alcohol.
3. The provider is positioned on the opposite side of the frown line to be treated, standing behind the head of the bed.
4. Attach a 30-gauge, ½-inch needle to the prefilled HA-lidocaine dermal filler syringe. Ensure that the needle is firmly affixed to the dermal filler syringe to prevent the needle popping off when plunger pressure is applied.
5. Prime the needle by depressing the syringe plunger until a small amount of dermal filler extrudes from the needle tip.
6. The first injection is started at the superior most portion of the frown line. Insert the needle at a 30-degree angle to the skin, direct it inferiorly, and advance to the needle hub. Apply gentle, constant pressure on the syringe plunger while gradually withdrawing needle to inject a linear thread of filler in the mid-dermis (Fig. 6).
7. If a second injection is required, the injection point is approximately one-needle length inferior to the first injection point and placed as above. Frown lines typically angle laterally, and the path of injection should follow the patient's specific frown line anatomy.

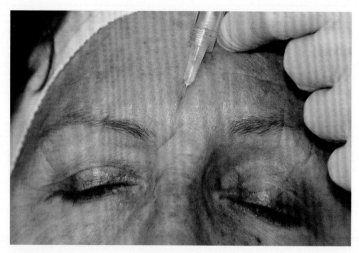

*FIGURE 6* ● Injection technique for dermal filler treatment of frown lines.

8. Compress the edges of the product placing both thumbs on either side of the frown line to mold the filler into the frown line.
9. Reposition and repeat the above injections for contralateral side of face.

## Tip

- Watch for tissue blanching and other ischemic signs or symptoms in the frown line area. If ischemia occurs, manage as described in Tissue Ischemia in the Complications section.

## Results

- Reduction of frown lines is immediately evident at the time of treatment. Figure 1 shows a 60-year-old woman with static frown lines before (A) and 2 weeks after (B) treatment with 0.3 mL HA-lidocaine dermal filler, Juvederm Ultra XC.

## Duration of Effects and Subsequent Treatments

- Visible correction of frown lines typically lasts 9 months to 1 year after treatment.
- Subsequent treatment with dermal filler is recommended when the volume of dermal filler product is visibly diminished and the frown lines become more prominent again prior to their pretreatment appearance.

## Follow-ups and Management

Patients are assessed 4 weeks after treatment to evaluate for reduction of frown lines. Common issues reported by patients include the following:

- **Bruising, swelling, erythema, and tenderness.** See Follow-ups and Management in the Introduction and Foundation Concepts section.
- **Persistent frown lines.** Persistent lines may be due to the following:
  - **Volume deficit.** Additional dermal filler may be necessary if a volume deficit persists. Typically, small volumes of 0.1–0.2 mL HA-lidocaine will achieve the desired result.

- **Dynamic frown lines.** Combination treatment with botulinum toxin may be required to achieve optimal reduction of frown lines with hyperdynamic musculature (see Combining Aesthetic Treatments later).
- **Superficial static lines.** These will typically soften over the subsequent months after patients have received botulinum toxin and dermal filler treatments. Resurfacing and collagen-stimulating procedures can further reduce static lines (see Combining Aesthetic Treatments later).

## Complications and Management

- General dermal filler complications and management are reviewed in the Complications section
- Tissue ischemia and necrosis
- Blindness

**Ischemia** and subsequent **tissue necrosis** in the frown line area can be due to either overfilling the tissue or vascular occlusion. It can present with or without pain and is usually visible as immediate blanching. Ischemia is managed urgently, as it can rapidly progress to tissue necrosis (see Complications section for management). **Blindness** due to retinal artery embolization following dermal filler treatment in the glabella has been reported.

## Combining Aesthetic Treatments and Maximizing Results

- **Botulinum toxin.** Combining dermal filler treatment of frown lines with botulinum toxin treatment of the glabellar complex muscles can improve reduction of frown lines. Botulinum toxin treatment of the glabellar complex is ideally performed 2 weeks prior to dermal filler treatment to relax hyperdynamic musculature; however, it may also be performed at the time of treatment, or after treatment once bruising and swelling resolve. In addition to softening static frown lines, reducing glabellar muscle contraction helps ensure the smoothest possible dermal filler results.
- **Skin resurfacing and collagen-stimulating treatments.** Reduction of superficial static frown lines can be improved by combining dermal fillers with skin resurfacing and collagen-stimulating procedures such as ablative and nonablative lasers, dermabrasion, and chemical peels. With the more aggressive procedures such as ablative and fractional ablative lasers, dermabrasion, and medium depth chemical peels, dermal filler treatments are performed after recovery. With less aggressive procedures such as nonablative lasers, superficial chemical peels, and microdermabrasion, dermal filler treatments may be performed during the same visit or prior to these procedures.

## Pricing

Dermal filler fees are based on the type of filler used, size and number of syringes, the injector's skill, and vary according to community pricing in different geographic regions. Prices range from $500 to 800 per syringe of 0.8 mL HA used for treatment of frown lines.

# Chapter 11

# Scars

### Rebecca Small, M.D.

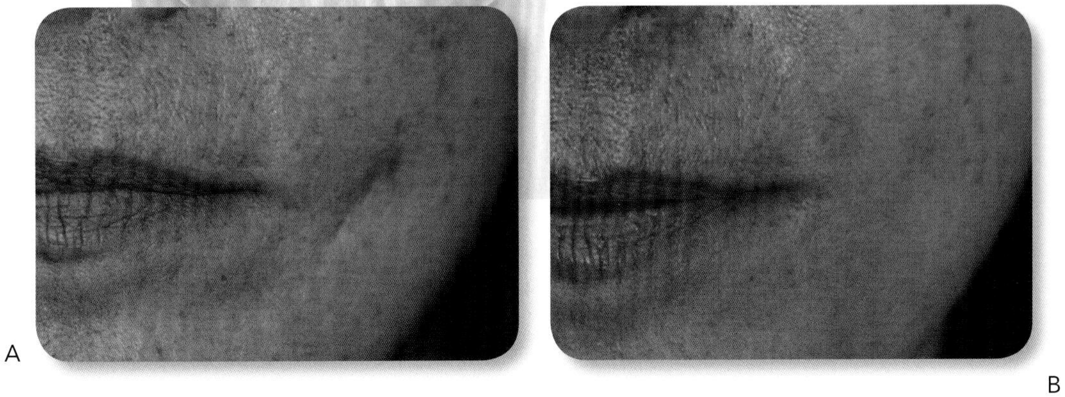

FIGURE 1 ● Scars before **(A)** and 4 weeks after **(B)** dermal filler treatment, using hyaluronic acid.

Atrophic depression scars on the face are common sequelae from skin excisions, acne, chickenpox and trauma. Soft, distensible scars can be effectively smoothed with dermal filler treatments.

## Indications

• Depression scars

## Anatomy

• **Wrinkles, folds, and contours.** Atrophic scars, or depression scars, typically present as either smooth scars with soft, rounded borders or deep, narrow ice pick scars. Histologically these scars are composed of fibrotic tissue, which can be tethered to the subcutaneous tissue.

## Patient Assessment

• Patient history is reviewed regarding the cause of scarring including acne, surgery, trauma, and infection. Discussion of expectations regarding the temporary nature of scar improvement with dermal filler treatments is important to ensure patient satisfaction.

- Scars are examined and the skin gently pulled, or distended, on either side using the first finger and thumb. Most atrophic scars with soft, rounded borders that are distensible can be improved with dermal fillers.

## Contraindications

- See Contraindications in the Introduction and Foundation Concepts section.
- Ice pick scars
- Nondistensible scars

## Treatment Goals

- Full effacement of depression scars without overfilling.

## Recommended Dermal Filler Product

- Basic hyaluronic acid (HA) dermal filler products lidocaine (HA-lidocaine) that have supple, soft tissue filling effects such as Juvederm® Ultra XC are recommended for treatment of depression scars. Other HA-lidocaine products may also be used such as Prevelle® Silk, however, this has a shorter duration of action (see Basic and Advanced Procedures in the Introduction and Foundation Concepts section).
- This chapter describes treatment of depression scars with Juvederm Ultra XC (HA-lidocaine).

## Dermal Filler Treatment Volumes

- The estimated HA dermal filler volume necessary for treatment is based on the extensiveness and depth of facial scarring. Small volumes are typically required for treatment of all facial scarring, which range from 0.3 to 0.4 mL HA-lidocaine.

## Equipment for Anesthesia

- General topical anesthetic supplies (see Equipment for Topical Anesthetics in the Anesthesia section)
- Benzocaine:lidocaine:tetracaine (BLT) ointment

## Equipment for Dermal Filler Procedure

- General dermal filler injection supplies (see Equipment for Topical Anesthetics in the Anesthesia section)
- 30-gauge, ½-inch needle
- Small wooden cotton-tipped applicators

## Anesthesia Overview

- **Topical anesthetic.** BLT may be used to achieve anesthesia for scars (see Topical Anesthetics in the Anesthesia section) as shown in Figure 2. HA dermal fillers formulated with lidocaine have improved patient tolerance relative to non-lidocaine

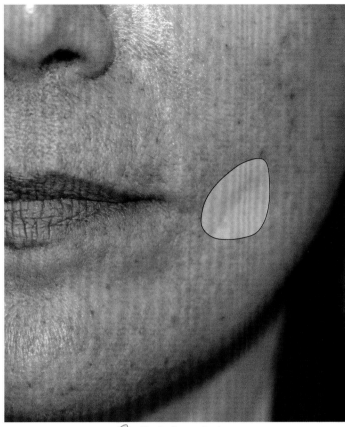

⬭ = Topical anesthetic

*FIGURE 2* ● Anesthesia for scar dermal filler treatment.

products and adequate anesthesia for scars can typically be obtained using a topical anesthetic.
- **Ice.** Ice is commonly used as an alternative to BLT in the scar area.

## Dermal Filler Procedure Overview

- **Overview.** An overview of injection points and injection technique for treatment of scars using a HA dermal filler is shown in Figure 3.
- **Number of injections.** Typically two to four fanning injections are performed based on the size of the scar (see Techniques for Dermal Filler Injection in the Introduction and Foundation Concepts section). Injection points are just outside the perimeter of the scar and opposite from each other.
- **Injection depth.** Dermal filler is injected in the superficial to mid-dermis for treatment of depression scars.
- **Cautions.** Ischemia and necrosis have been reported with injection of scars due to overfilling of tissue or vascular occlusion. Using thin dermal filler products, intradermal placement, low filler volumes, gentle plunger pressure, and keeping the needle slowly moving at all times in a retrograde fashion while injecting may reduce the likelihood of vascular compromise.

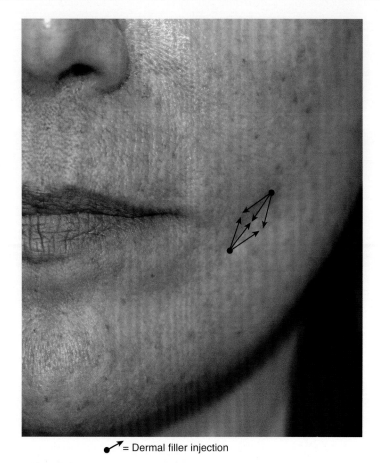

= Dermal filler injection

*FIGURE 3* ● Overview of depression scar dermal filler injections.

## Performing the Procedure: Dermal Filler Treatment of Scars

### Anesthesia

1. Clean and prepare the scar area with alcohol.
2. Apply ½ g BLT as a thin layer to the scar areas using a cotton-tipped applicator or gloved finger (Fig. 2). Gently rub the BLT using small circular motions to enhance penetration into the skin. Occlusion with plastic wrap is not necessary.
3. Remove BLT 15–30 minutes after application using alcohol.

### Dermal Filler

1. Position the patient in a 60-degree reclined position.
2. Prepare the scars with alcohol.
3. The provider is positioned on the same side as the scar to be injected.
4. Attach a 30-gauge, ½-inch needle to the prefilled HA-lidocaine dermal filler syringe. Ensure that the needle is firmly affixed to the dermal filler syringe to prevent the needle popping off when plunger pressure is applied.

5. Prime the needle by depressing the syringe plunger until a small amount of dermal filler extrudes from the needle tip.
6. Choose a side of the scar for the first fanning injection. Insert the needle just outside the perimeter of the scar at a 15-degree angle to the skin, and advance the needle until the tip reaches the midline of the scar. Apply firm and constant pressure on the syringe plunger while gradually withdrawing needle to inject a linear thread of filler in the superficial to mid-dermis. Without fully withdrawing the needle from the skin, fan the needle clockwise using small angulations to ensure dermal filler placement is contiguous (see Techniques for Dermal Filler Injection in the Introduction and Foundation Concepts section). Repeat until desired correction is achieved.
7. The second injection point is opposite the first, and dermal filler is injected as described above.
8. For larger scars, third and fourth injections may be required and are opposite to one another at 90 degrees to the above injections.
9. Smooth the scar and the perimeter of the scar using the first finger intraorally and a cotton-tipped applicator extraorally to compress any visible or palpable bumps of filler product.

## Tips

- Dermal filler can collect around the margin of some scars. If this is evident, discontinue injection, smooth the filler, and resume injecting from another point around the perimeter of the scar.
- The gray needle tip should not be visible through the skin. If this is observed, the needle is too superficial and should be redirected slightly deeper in the dermis without being fully withdrawn from the skin.
- Watch for tissue blanching and other ischemic signs or symptoms with scar injections. If ischemia occurs, manage as described in the Complications section.

## Results

- Reduction of scars is immediately evident at the time of treatment. Figure 1 shows a 50-year-old woman with scarring from previous autologous fat injection for cheek hollows, before (A) and 4 weeks after (B), treatment with 0.2-mL HA-lidocaine dermal filler, Juvederm Ultra XC.

## Duration of Effects and Subsequent Treatments

- Visible correction of scars typically lasts 6–9 months after treatment.
- Subsequent treatment with dermal filler is recommended when the volume of dermal filler product is visibly diminished and scars become more prominent again, prior to their pretreatment appearance.

## Follow-Ups and Management

Patients are assessed 4 weeks after treatment to evaluate for reduction of scars. Common issues reported by patients during this time include the following:

- **Bruising, swelling, erythema, and tenderness.** See Follow-Ups and Management in the Introduction and Foundation Concepts section.

- **Persistent scars.** Additional dermal filler may be necessary if a volume deficit persists. Typically 0.1–0.2 mL HA-lidocaine will achieve the desired result.

## Complications and Management

- General dermal filler complications and management are reviewed in the Complications section
- Bumpiness

   **Bumpiness** can be visible if scars are not manually smoothed after treatment. If bumps are visible at the follow-up visit, compress as directed earlier.

## Combining Aesthetic Treatments and Maximizing Results

- **Skin resurfacing and collagen stimulating treatments.** Reduction of superficial depression scars can be improved by combining dermal fillers with skin resurfacing or collagen stimulating procedures such as ablative and nonablative lasers, dermabrasion, and chemical peels. With the more aggressive procedures such as ablative and fractional ablative lasers, dermabrasion, and medium-depth chemical peels, dermal filler treatments are performed after recovery. With less aggressive procedures such as nonablative lasers, superficial chemical peels, and microdermabrasion, dermal filler treatments may be performed in the same visit or prior to these procedures.
- **Dermatologic surgery.** Results with poorly distensible scars can be improved when combining subcision, whereby the fibrotic attachments to deeper tissues are released using a specialized blade or large gauge needle, with dermal filler treatment afterward.

## Pricing

Dermal filler fees are based on the type of filler used, size and number of syringes, the injector's skill, and vary according to community pricing in different geographic regions. Prices range from $500 to $800 per syringe of 0.8 mL HA for treatment of scars.

**Chapter 12**

# Layering Dermal Fillers (Moderate to Severe Nasolabial Folds)

Rebecca Small, M.D.

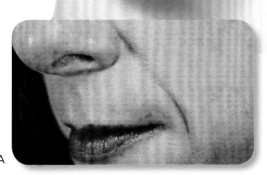

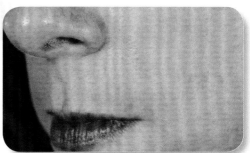

A

B

*FIGURE 1* ● Nasolabial fold before **(A)** and 4 weeks after **(B)** dermal filler treatment layering calcium hydroxylapatite and hyaluronic acid.

When treating facial areas that exhibit moderate to severe volume loss such as the nasolabial folds, marionette lines, and mental crease, improved outcomes can often be achieved by layering two types of dermal filler products. With this technique, a dermal filler with more structural support is used to provide a foundation in areas of deep dermal volume loss, and a thinner, more malleable dermal filler is overlaid to smooth superficial fine lines and wrinkles. These more complex layering techniques are considered advanced dermal filler treatments. Treatment of moderate to severe nasolabial folds is used in this chapter to illustrate the dermal filler layering technique.

## Indications

• Moderate to severe nasolabial folds

## Anatomy

• **Wrinkles, folds, and contours.** Nasolabial folds, or melolabial folds, course diagonally in the midface from the nasal ala toward the corner of the lip (see Dermal Filler

151

Anatomy, Figs. 1 and 2). The lateral nasal artery is the main vascular supply for the nasal tip and ala, and is in close proximity to the nasolabial fold, 2–3 mm superior to the nasal alar groove (see Dermal Filler Anatomy, Figs. 3 and 5).

## Patient Assessment

- Patients with moderate to severe nasolabial folds are assessed for areas of deep volume loss, visible as concave contours, and superficial wrinkles. Patients with both of these findings typically achieve the best results with dermal filler treatments using the layering technique outlined in this chapter.
- Patients presenting with excess laxity and hanging skin folds usually require surgical intervention for significant improvement.
- Patients with nasolabial folds may also have volume deficits in the malar area. If significant malar flattening is present, it is advisable to perform malar augmentation first and reassess nasolabial folds at the follow-up visit. Restoring midface volume often reduces nasolabial folds and smaller treatment volumes for the nasolabial folds may be required after malar augmentation is performed (see Malar Augmentation chapter).

## Contraindications

- See Contraindications in the Introduction and Foundation Concepts section.

## Treatment Goals

- Reduction of nasolabial folds without full effacement.

## Recommended Dermal Filler Product

- Areas of deep volume loss are ideally treated with dermal filler products that offer more structural support such as Radiesse® or Perlane-L® (see Basic and Advanced Procedures in the Introduction and Foundation Concepts section).
- Superficial lines are ideally treated with thinner, more supple dermal filler products such as Juvederm® Ultra XC or Prevelle Silk® (see Basic and Advanced Procedures in the Introduction and Foundation Concepts section).
- This chapter describes layering treatment of nasolabial folds with the following products:
  - **Deep volume loss areas** are treated with Radiesse, a calcium hydroxylapatite (CaHA) filler. CaHA is mixed with lidocaine (CaHA-lidocaine).
  - **Superficial lines** are treated with Juvederm Ultra XC (hyaluronic acid-lidocaine).

## Dermal Filler Treatment Volumes

- The estimated dermal filler volume necessary for treatment is based on patients' observed facial anatomy and volume loss in the treatment area.
- Layering for treatment of moderate to severe nasolabial folds typically requires a total volume of 1.2–1.6 mL CaHA-lidocaine (Radiesse).

- Layering for treatment of moderate to severe nasolabial folds typically requires a total volume of 0.6–0.8 mL HA-lidocaine (Juvederm Ultra XC).

## Equipment for Anesthesia

- Local infiltration injection supplies (see Equipment for Injectable Anesthetics in the Anesthesia section)
- Lidocaine HCl 2% with epinephrine 1:100,000 buffered (referred to as buffered 2% lidocaine-epinephrine solution)
- 30 gauge, ½ inch needle

## Equipment for Dermal Filler Procedure

- General dermal filler injection supplies (see Equipment in the Introduction and Foundation Concepts section)
- CaHA mixing supplies (see Equipment in the Introduction and Foundation Concepts section)
- 27-gauge, 1-¼ inch needle for CaHA-lidocaine
- 30-gauge ½-inch needle for HA-lidocaine

## Anesthesia Overview

- **Local lidocaine infiltration.** Buffered 2% lidocaine-epinephrine solution can be used to achieve anesthesia for nasolabial folds. Both folds are anesthetized using six injections of 0.1 mL for a total volume of 0.6 mL (Fig. 2).

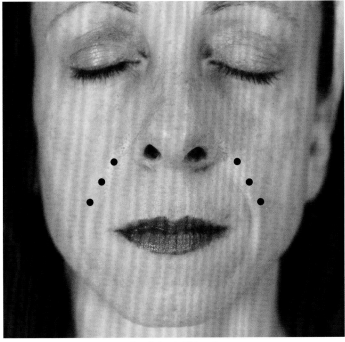

● = 0.1 mL Lidocaine

*FIGURE 2* ● Anesthesia for nasolabial fold dermal filler treatment.

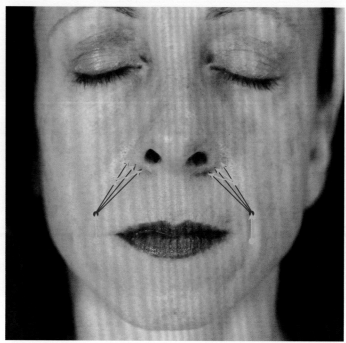

●——▶ = Calcium hydroxylapatite dermal filler       ✐ = Hyaluronic acid dermal filler

*FIGURE 3* ● Overview of nasolabial fold dermal filler layering technique.

- See the Injectable Anesthetics in the Anesthesia chapter for additional information on local infiltration methods. Sensitivity increases with proximity to the nose and injections are started at the inferior portion of the fold.

## Dermal Filler Procedure Overview

- **Overview.** An overview of injection points and techniques for layering dermal fillers in the nasolabial folds, using CaHA-lidocaine and HA-lidocaine, is shown in Figure 3. First, dermal filler products with more structural support (CaHA-lidocaine) are injected in areas of deep volume loss. More supple dermal filler products (HA-lidocaine) are then used to smooth superficial wrinkles, typically in the superior and inferior portions of the nasolabial folds.
- **CaHA-lidocaine preparation** is performed at the time of treatment (see Calcium Hydroxylapatite and Lidocaine Preparations in the Introduction and Foundation Concepts section).
- **Number of injections and injection depth** (see Techniques for Dermal Filler Injection in the Introduction and Foundation Concepts section).
  - **For CaHA-lidocaine,** there is one fanning injection per side of the face and injections are placed in the deep dermis.
  - **For HA-lidocaine,** there is typically one fanning injection for the superior portion, and one linear thread injection for the inferior portion of the nasolabial fold on each side of the face. Injections are placed in the superficial to mid-dermis.
- **Cautions.** The lateral nasal artery is the main vascular supply for the nasal tip and ala, and is avoided with treatment of nasolabial folds.

# Performing the Procedure: Dermal Filler Layering for Nasolabial Folds

## Anesthesia

1. Clean and prepare the skin lateral to the nasolabial folds with alcohol.
2. Inject buffered 2% lidocaine-epinephrine solution subcutaneously as shown in Figure 2.
3. Allow a few minutes for anesthesia.

## Dermal Filler for Deep Volume Loss—Calcium Hydroxylapatite

1. Position the patient in a 60-degree reclined position.
2. Clean and prepare the skin of the nasolabial folds with alcohol.
3. The provider is positioned on the same side as the nasolabial fold to be injected.
4. Attach a 27-gauge, 1¼-inch needle to the prepared CaHA-lidocaine dermal filler syringe. Ensure that the needle is firmly affixed to the dermal filler syringe to prevent the needle popping off when plunger pressure is applied.
5. Prime the needle by depressing the syringe plunger until a small amount of dermal filler extrudes from the needle tip.
6. Determine the first insertion point by laying the needle just medial to the nasolabial fold such that the needle tip is 1 mm below the nasal ala. The first injection point is at the needle hub (Fig. 4).
7. Insert the needle at a 30-degree angle to the skin, directing it superiorly toward the nasal ala and advance to the needle hub. Apply firm and constant pressure on the syringe

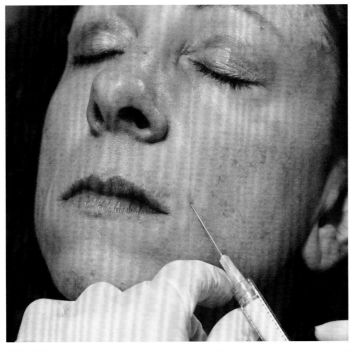

**FIGURE 4** ● Calcium hydroxylapatite needle insertion for treatment of the nasolabial folds.

plunger while gradually withdrawing needle to inject a linear thread of filler in the deep dermis just medial to the nasolabial fold. Without fully withdrawing the needle from the skin, fan the needle inferomedially, using small angulations to ensure dermal filler placement is contiguous (Figs. 5A and 5B). Repeat until desired correction is achieved.

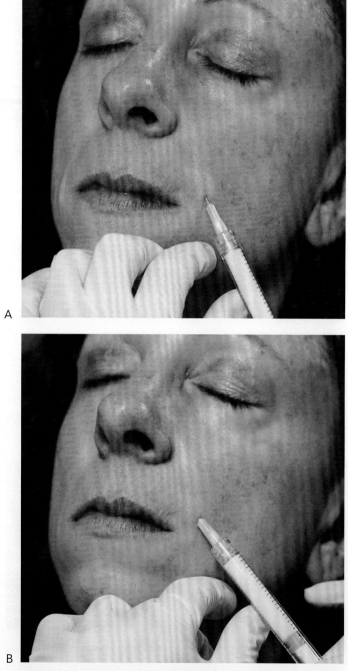

**FIGURE 5** ● Calcium hydroxylapatite for treatment of the nasolabial folds: fanning from **(A)** to **(B)**.

8. Compress the treatment areas with one finger intraorally and the thumb on the skin, using firm pressure to smooth any visible or palpable bumps of filler product.
9. Reposition to the opposite side and repeat the above injection for the other nasolabial fold.

### Dermal Filler for Superficial Lines—Hyaluronic Acid

1. Repeat steps 1–3 as described above.
2. Attach a 30-gauge, ½-inch needle to the prefilled HA-lidocaine dermal filler syringe. Ensure that the needle is firmly affixed to the dermal filler syringe to prevent the needle popping off when plunger pressure is applied.
3. Prime the needle by depressing the syringe plunger until a small amount of dermal filler extrudes from the needle tip.
4. For the superior portion of the nasolabial fold, the needle insertion point is one needle length inferior to the nasal ala, just medial to the nasolabial fold. Insert the needle at a 30-degree angle to the skin, directing it superiorly toward the nasal ala and advance to the needle hub. Apply firm and constant pressure on the syringe plunger while gradually withdrawing needle to inject a linear thread of filler in the superficial dermis just medial to the nasolabial fold; without fully withdrawing the needle from the skin, fan the needle inferomedially, using small angulations to ensure dermal filler placement is contiguous (Figs. 6A and 6B). Repeat until desired correction is achieved.
5. Compress the treatment areas with one finger intraorally and the thumb on the skin, using firm pressure to smooth any visible or palpable bumps of filler product.
6. For the inferior portion of the nasolabial fold, the needle insertion point is at the inferior end of the nasolabial fold. Insert the needle at a 30-degree angle to the skin, directing it superiorly toward the nasal ala and advance to the needle hub. Apply firm and constant pressure on the syringe plunger while gradually withdrawing needle to inject a linear thread of filler in the superficial dermis (Fig. 7).
7. Reposition to the opposite side and repeat the above injections for the other nasolabial fold.

## Tips

- Avoid placing CaHA in the superficial dermis as this may result in an undesirable visible ridge of filler which does not readily compress.
- Avoid treating lateral to the nasolabial folds as this can exacerbate the folds.
- Watch for tissue blanching or other ischemic signs and symptoms. If ischemia occurs, manage as described in the Complications section.

## Results

- Reduction of nasolabial folds is immediately evident at the time of treatment. Figure 8 shows a 46-year-old woman with severe nasolabial folds immediately after dermal filler layering treatment of the left half of the face. Dermal filler volumes for treatment of both nasolabial folds were 1.5 mL CaHA-lidocaine (Radiesse) and 0.8-mL HA (Juvederm Ultra Plus). Figure 1 shows the same patient before (A) and 4 weeks after (B) the layering treatment.

## Duration of Effects and Subsequent Treatments

- CaHA dermal filler typically lasts 18 months and HA dermal filler typically lasts 6 months to 1 year.

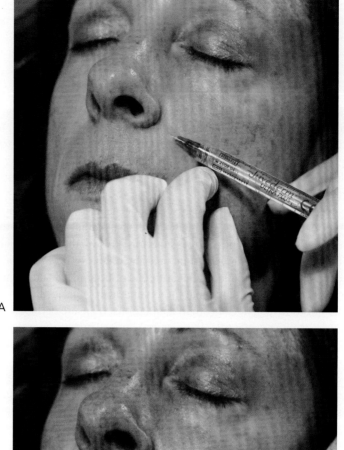

*FIGURE 6* ● Hyaluronic acid layering for treatment of the superior nasolabial folds: fanning from **(A)** to **(B)**.

- Subsequent treatment with dermal filler is recommended when the volume of dermal filler product is visibly diminished and the nasolabial folds are more evident, prior to their pretreatment appearance. With layering of dermal fillers in the nasolabial folds, a subsequent treatment with HA dermal filler only is typically performed at 6–9 months.

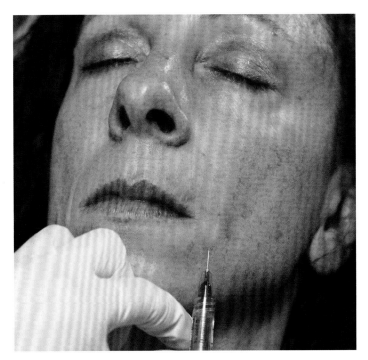

FIGURE 7 ● Hyaluronic acid treatment of the inferior nasolabial fold.

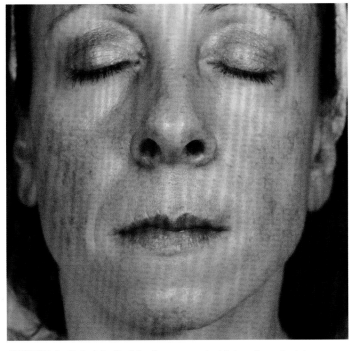

FIGURE 8 ● Left half of the face treated with layering of calcium hydroxylapatite and hyaluronic acid dermal fillers.

## Follow-Ups and Management

Patients are assessed 4 weeks after treatment to evaluate for reduction of the nasolabial folds. Common issues reported by patients during this time include the following:

- **Bruising, swelling, erythema, and tenderness.** See Follow-up section for recommendations and management strategies in the Introduction and Foundation Concepts section.
- **Persistent nasolabial folds.** Patients should be assessed for the following:
  - **Static nasolabial folds.** Additional dermal filler may be necessary if a volume deficit persists. Typically 0.4–0.8 mL HA-lidocaine will achieve the desired result.
  - **Dynamic nasolabial folds.** Combination treatment with botulinum toxin may be required to achieve optimal results in patients with deep dynamic nasolabial folds, see Combining Aesthetic Treatments later.

## Complications and Management

- General dermal filler complications and management are reviewed in the Complications section
- Tissue ischemia and tissue necrosis

   **Tissue ischemia** resulting from intravascular injection and occlusion of the angular artery may occur with nasolabial fold treatments. Signs of vascular compromise and ischemia include a violaceous reticular pattern or white blanching, and may be painful or painless. These changes may be seen on the nose and/or nasolabial fold, and can present immediately, or be delayed. One case report identified ischemic changes 6 hours after dermal filler treatment. Ischemia is managed urgently as it can rapidly progress to **tissue necrosis** (see Complications section).

## Combining Aesthetic Treatments and Maximizing Results

- **Botulinum toxin.** Some patients have excessive contraction of the lip levator muscles during smiling, resulting in deep nasolabial folds and a "gummy" smile. In these patients, combining dermal filler treatment of the nasolabial fold with botulinum toxin treatment of the levator labii superioris alaeque nasi muscle can improve reduction of nasolabial folds.
- **Dermal filler in adjacent areas.** Patients requiring nasolabial fold treatment may also have volume deficits in the malar area. It is advisable to perform malar augmentation first and reassess nasolabial folds at the follow-up visit (see Malar Augmentation chapter).

## Pricing

Dermal filler fees are based on the type of filler used, size and number of syringes, the injector's skill, and vary according to community pricing in different geographic regions. Prices range from $500 to $800 per syringe of 0.8 mL HA and $650 to $1200 per syringe of 1.5 mL CaHA for layering treatment of nasolabial folds with moderate to severe volume loss.

# Aesthetic Intake Form

Date:_____

NAME: _____ AGE:_____ * Date of Birth:_____

      Last,      First

ADDRESS: _____ CITY:_____ ZIP: _____

MOBILE PHONE: _____ ☐ OK TO CONTACT ☐ LEAVE MESSAGE HERE

HOME PHONE: _____ ☐ OK TO CONTACT ☐ LEAVE MESSAGE HERE

WORK PHONE: _____ ☐ OK TO CONTACT ☐ LEAVE MESSAGE HERE

E-MAIL: _____ ☐ OK TO CONTACT

OCCUPATION: _____ How did you hear about us?: _____

In order of importance, beginning with 1, please rank what you would like to see improved in your skin:
_____ Reduction of wrinkles and fine lines _____ Reduction of brown spots/sun damage _____ Reduction of oil/acne _____ Reduction of hair _____ Reduction of redness _____ Tattoo removal _____ Other: _____
_____

| Medical History | Yes | No | Please check all medical conditions past or present | Yes | No |
|---|---|---|---|---|---|
| Are you or is it possible that you may be pregnant? | | | Keloid scarring | | |
| Are you breastfeeding? | | | Cold sores | | |
| Do you form thick or raised scars from cuts or burns? | | | Herpes (genital) | | |
| After injury to the skin (such as cuts/burns) do you have: | | | Easy bruising or bleeding | | |
|     Darkening of the skin in that area (hyperpigmentation) <br>     Lightening of the skin in that area (hypopigmentation) | | | Active skin infection | | |
| Hair removal by plucking, waxing, electrolysis or depilatory creams in the last 4 weeks? | | | Moles that have recently changed, itched, or bled | | |
| Tanning (tanning bed) or sun expose in the last 4 weeks? | | | Recent increase in amount of hair | | |
| Tanning products or spray on tan in the last 2 weeks? | | | Asthma | | |
| Do you have a tan now in the area to be treated? | | | Seasonal allergies/allergic rhinitis | | |

*(Continued)*

| Medical History | Yes | No | Please check all medical conditions past or present | Yes | No |
|---|---|---|---|---|---|
| Do you use sunscreen daily with SPF 30 or higher? | | | Eczema | | |
| Have you ever had a skin cancer? | | | Thyroid imbalance | | |
| List your common outdoor activities: | | | Poor healing | | |
| Have you ever had a photosensitive disorder? (e.g. Lupus) | | | Diabetes | | |
| Do you have a personal history of seizures? | | | Heart condition | | |
| Permanent make-up or tattoos? | | | High blood pressure | | |
| Have you used Accutane in the last 6 months? | | | Pacemaker | | |
| Are you currently taking any antibiotics? Which: | | | Disease of nerves or muscles (e.g. ALS, Myasthenia gravis, Lambert-Eaton or other) | | |
| Are you using Retin-A or Glycolic products? | | | Cancer | | |
| What is the name of your regular physician: | | | HIV/AIDS | | |
| Do you have an allergy or sensitivity to lidocaine, latex, sulfa medications, hydroquinone, aloe, bee stings? (circle) | | | Autoimmune disease (e.g. rheumatoid arthritis, Scleroderma) | | |
| Life threatening allergy to anything? | | | Hepatitis | | |
| Do you currently smoke? | | | Shingles | | |
| Do you have scars on the face? | | | Migraine headaches | | |
| Explanation of items marked "Yes": | | | Other illness, health problems or medical conditions not listed: | | |

\* For minors, please request Guardian information form.

I certify that the information I have given is complete and accurate. _____Initials _____ Staff initials

**For Internal Use Only Below This Line**

_____

_____

_____

_____

# Before and After Instructions for Dermal Filler Treatments

## Before Treatment

- Avoid aspirin (any product containing acetylsalicylic acid), vitamin E, St John's Wort, and other dietary supplements including: ginkgo, evening primrose oil, garlic, feverfew, and ginseng for 2 weeks.
- Avoid ibuprofen (Advil, Motrin) and alcohol for 2 days.
- If possible, come to your appointment with a cleanly washed face without make-up.

## After Treatment

- Skin redness and swelling in the treatment area is common. This should resolve within a few days. If it persists longer than 3 days, please contact your physician.
- Do not massage the treated areas.
- Avoid applying heat to the treated area until any swelling or bruising have resolved. Routine washing and showering is fine.
- Avoid activities that cause facial flushing on the day of treatment including: consuming alcohol, exercising, and tanning.
- Gently apply a cool compress or wrapped ice pack to the treated areas for 15 minutes every few hours as needed to reduce discomfort, swelling, or bruising up to a few days after treatment. If bruising occurs it typically resolves within 7–10 days.
- After treatment, oral and/or topical Arnica montana may help reduce bruising and swelling.
- If 2–4 weeks after treatment you feel that you require a touch-up, please contact your physician.

# Consent for Dermal Filler Treatments

Dermal fillers are used for the treatment of facial creases, wrinkles, folds, contour defects, depression scars, facial lipoatrophy (loss of fat), and enhancement purposes. These treatments involve multiple injections of filler into or below the skin to fill wrinkles and restore volume. The effects of dermal fillers are temporary and no guarantees can be made regarding how long correction will last in a specific patient.

Alternatives to temporary fillers include, but are not limited to: permanent dermal fillers, laser resurfacing and skin tightening, surgical face-lift, or no treatment at all.

Possible risks, side-effects, and complications with dermal fillers include, but are not limited to:

- Bruising, redness, and swelling
- Visible raised areas or bumpiness at/around the treated site
- Asymmetry, overcorrection, or undercorrection
- Unpredictable persistence of filler, either shorter or longer than anticipated
- Prolonged discoloration of the skin such as brown, grayish, bluish, or reddish coloration
- Filler material may be extruded from the skin in rare cases
- Prolonged or severe swelling
- Infection
- Rarely granulomas or firm nodules may form
- Benign tumor formation (keratoacanthomas)
- Allergic reaction with itchiness, redness, and in extremely rare cases generalized allergic response such as whole body swelling, respiratory problems, and shock
- Scarring is extremely rare
- Skin breakdown or ulceration
- Blindness

A remote and rare risk is that of filler injection into a blood vessel (blood vessel occlusion) or overfilling tissue that can block blood flow to the treated area or to distant areas, causing tissue damage and tissue death (necrosis), which can be seen as skin breakdown or ulceration. Blood vessel occlusion near the eye can result in blindness.

The administration of anesthetics may be necessary or advisable in association with dermal filler treatments to reduce pain. This includes, but is not limited to: local anesthetic such as anesthetic injections with lidocaine 1–2% with or without epinephrine; and/or topical anesthetics such as benzocaine/lidocaine/tetracaine; and/or topical oral benzocaine preparations. Complications of these anesthetics include, but are not limited to: skin irritation (itching or redness), lightheadedness, rapid heart rate, visual disturbance, tongue numbness, and seizure.

Photographs taken shall be part of the medical record and used for documentation of response to treatment.

My signature below certifies that I have fully read this consent form and understand the written information provided to me regarding the proposed procedure. I have been adequately informed about the procedure including: the potential benefits, risks, limitations, and alternative treatments, and I have had all questions and concerns answered to my satisfaction.

Patient Name _____

Patient Signature _____          Date _____

# Dermal Filler Procedure Notes

Name: _____     DOB:_____

| Date: | | Yes | No |
|---|---|---|---|
| Changes in medications/allergies? | | * | |
| Pregnant or nursing? | | | |
| Changes in health status? | | ** | |

**Procedure:** ☐ Prepped site with alcohol
☐ Lidocaine 1%/2% with/without epinephrine buffered/not buffered was injected using a 30G ½ inch needle.
  ☐ SQ in 0.1 ml amounts adjacent to tx area for a total of _____ mL
  ☐ Intraoral lip mucosa in 0.1 ml amounts for a total of _____ mL
  ☐ Intraoral upper lip ring block injections in 2 sites: lateral to the frenulum and lateral to the canine tooth, submucosal at the gingivobuccal margin, for atotal of _____ mL bilaterally.
  ☐ Intraoral lower lip ring block injections in 2 sites: lateral to the frenulum and lateral to the first bicuspid tooth, submucosal at the gingivobuccal margin, for a total of _____mL
☐ Topical anesthetic: BLT _____ g for _____mins
Type of dermal filler used: ☐ _____ , volume_____ mL
                            ☐ _____ , volume_____ mL

S O  S= Subjective O= Objective
☐ ☐ Smile lines/ Nasolabial folds
☐ ☐ Vertical lip lines
☐ ☐ Marionette lines/Downturned corners of mouth
☐ ☐ Lip enhancement: ☐ body ☐ border ☐ upper ☐ lower
☐ ☐ Other:_____

**Pre-procedure:**
☐ R/B/C/A for procedure discussed and all questions answered.
☐ Written pre and post tx instructions given to patient and reviewed.
☐ Consent signed in chart.
☐ Photos taken:   Yes/No
☐ Other:_____

**Post-procedure:**
☐ Patient tolerated procedure_____
☐ Bruise noted_____
☐ Applied cold compress to reduce swelling.

        Last,                    First

A/P: Contour defect/volume loss_____ (areas)

Notes: _____
_____
_____
_____

*See Medication and Allergy List **See below
☐ See narrative progress notes          **Performed by:** _____

| Date: | | Yes | No |
|---|---|---|---|
| Changes in medications/allergies? | | * | |
| Pregnant or nursing? | | | |
| Changes in health status? | | ** | |

**Procedure:** ☐ Prepped site with alcohol
☐ Lidocaine 1%/2% with/without epinephrine buffered/not buffered was injected using a 30G ½ inch needle.
  ☐ SQ in 0.1ml amounts adjacent to tx area for a total of _____ mL
  ☐ Intraoral lip mucosa in 0.1 ml amounts for a total of _____ mL
  ☐ Intraoral upper lip ring block injections in 2 sites: lateral to the frenulum and lateral to the canine tooth, submucosal at the gingivobuccal margin, for a total of _____ mL bilaterally.
  ☐ Intraoral lower lip ring block injections in 2 sites: lateral to the frenulum and lateral to the first bicuspid tooth, submucosal at the gingivobuccal margin, for atotal of _____mL
☐ Topical anesthetic: BLT _____ g for _____mins
Type of dermal filler used: ☐_____ , volume_____ mL
                            ☐_____ , volume_____ mL

S O  S= Subjective O= Objective
☐ ☐ Smile lines/ Nasolabial folds
☐ ☐ Vertical lip lines
☐ ☐ Marionette lines/Cornersof mouth
☐ ☐ Lip enhancement: ☐ body ☐ border ☐ upper ☐ lower
☐ ☐ Other: _____

**Pre-procedure:**
☐ R/B/C/A for procedure discussed and all questions ans.
☐ Written pre and post tx instructions given to patient and reviewed.
☐ Consent signed in chart.
☐ Photos taken: Yes/No
☐ Other:_____

**Post-procedure:**
☐ Patient tolerated procedure_____
☐ Bruise noted_____
☐ Applied cold compressto reduce swelling.

A/P: Contour defect/volume loss_____ (areas)

Notes: _____
_____
_____
_____

*See Medication and Allergy List **See below
☐ See narrative progress notes          **Performed by:** _____

# Supply Sources

**Dermal Fillers**

Allergan (Juvederm®)
Phone: 1-800-377-7790
www.allergan.com

Bioform Medical/Merz (Radiesse®)
Phone: 1-650-286-4000
www.bioform.com

Medicis Aesthetics (Restylane®, Perlane®)
Phone: 1-866-222-1480
www.medicis.com

Mentor (Prevelle® Silk)
Phone: 1-866-250-5115
www.mentorcorp.com

**Hyaluronidase**

Amphastar Pharmaceuticals (Amphadase®)
Phone: 1-800-423-4136
www.amphastar.com

Ista Pharmaceuticals (Vitrase®)
Phone: 1-949-788-6000
www.istavision.com/products/vitrase.html

**Topical Anesthetics**

American Health Solutions Pharmacy (BLT ointment which contains benzocaine 20%/
lidocaine 6%/tetracaine 4%)
Phone: 1-310-838-7422

APP Pharmaceuticals (EMLA® which contains lidocaine 2.5%/ prilocaine 2.5%)
Phone: 1-847-413-2075
www.apppharma.com

PharmaDerm (L-M-X®  which contains lidocaine 4%–5%)
Phone: 1-973-514-4240
www.pharmaderm.com

Ultradent Products (Ultracare® gel which contains benzocaine 20%)
Phone: 1-800-552-5512
www.ultradent.com

J. Morita USA (CaineTips® which contains benzocaine 20%)
Phone: 1-888-566-7482
www.jmoritausa.com

**Cooling Products**
ThermoTek (ArTek Spot™ contact cooling device)
Phone: 1-972-874-4949
www.thermotek.com

Gebauer Company (Pain Ease® vapocoolant spray)
Phone: 1-800-321-9348
www.gebauer.com

**General Injection Supplies**
McKesson
Phone: 1-800-446-3008
www.mckesson.com

**Make-up for Bruises**
Jane Iredale (Corrective Colors®)
Phone: 1-800-762-1132
www.janeiredale.com

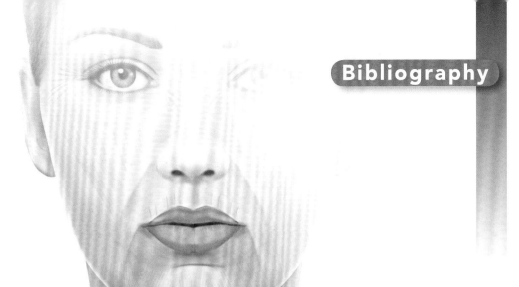

## Aesthetic Procedure Statistics and Overview

Cosmetic Surgery National Data Bank Statistics. American Society for Aesthetic Plastic Surgery. http://www.surgery.org/media/statistics.

Fedok FG. Advances in minimally invasive facial rejuvenation. Current Opin Otolaryngol Head Neck Surg. 2008;16(4):359–368.

Small R. Aesthetic procedures in office practice. Am Fam Physician. 2009;80(11):1231–1237.

## Consultation

Small R. Aesthetic Principles and Consultation. In: Usatine R, Pfenninger J, Stuhlberg D, Small R, eds. Dermatologic and Cosmetic Procedures in Office Practice. Philadelphia, PA. Elsevier. 2011;230–240.

Small R. Aesthetic Procedures Introduction. In: Mayeaux E, ed. The Essential Guide to Primary Care Procedures. Philadelphia, PA. Lippincott Williams & Wilson. 2009;195–199.

## Facial Anatomy

Goldberg RA. The three periorbital hollows: a paradigm for periorbital rejuvenation. Plast Reconstr Surg. 2005;116(6):1796–1804.

Netter FH. Atlas of Human Anatomy. 4th Edn. Philadelphia, PA. Saunders. 2006; 24, 25, 35–50.

## Dermal Fillers General

Alam M, Gladstone H, Kramer EM, et al. ASDS guidelines of care: injectable fillers. Dermatol Surg. 2008;34(Suppl 1):S115–S148.

Elson M. Dermal Fillers. In: Pfenninger JL, Folwer GC, eds. Procedures for Primary Care, 3rd ed. Mosby/Elsevier, Philadelphia, PA, 2011;373–378.

Fagien S, Klein AW. A brief overview and history of temporary fillers: evolution, advantages, and limitations. Plast Reconstr Surg. 2007;120(6 Suppl):8S–16S.

Goldman MP. Optimizing the use of fillers for facial rejuvenation: the right tool for the right job. Cosmetic Dermatology. 2007;20(7 S3):14–26.

Narins RS, Donofrio LM. Update on Fillers. Dermatol Surg. 2010;36:729.

Niamtu J. Facial aging and regional enhancement with injectable fillers. Cosmetic Dermatology. 2007; 20(5 Suppl):S14–S20.

Sadick NS. Soft tissue augmentation: selection, mode of operation, and proper use of injectable agents. Cosmetic Dermatology. 2007;20(5 S2):8–13.

Small R. Dermal Fillers. In: Usatine R, Pfenninger J, Stuhlberg D, Small R, eds. Dermatologic and Cosmetic Procedures in Office Practice. Philadelphia, PA. Elsevier. 2011;298–308.

Small R. Dermal Fillers for Facial Rejuvenation. In: Mayeaux E, ed. The Essential Guide to Primary Care Procedures. Philadelphia, PA. Lippincott Williams & Wilson. 2009;214–233.

Werschler WP, Kane M. Optimal use of facial filling agents: understanding the products. Cosmetic Dermatology. 2007;20(5 Suppl):S4–S47.

## Hyaluronic Acid Dermal Fillers

Andre P. New trends in face rejuvenation by hyaluronic acid injections. J Cosmet Dermatol. 2008;7(4):251–258.

Born T. Hyaluronic acids. Clin Plast Surg. 2006;33(4):525–538.

Brandt F, Bank D, Cross SL, et al. A lidocaine-containing formulation of large-gel particle hyaluronic acid alleviates pain. Dermatol Surg. 2010;36(Suppl 3):1876–1885.

Carruthers J, Carruthers A, Tezel A, et al. Volumizing with a 20-mg/mL smooth, highly cohesive, viscous hyaluronic acid filler and its role in facial rejuvenation therapy. Dermatol Surg. 2010;36(Suppl 3):1886–1892.

Dover JS, Rubin MG, Bhatia AC. Review of the efficacy, durability, and safety data of two nonanimal stabilized hyaluronic acid fillers from a prospective, randomized, comparative, multicenter study. Dermatol Surg. 2009;35(Suppl 1):322–330.

Green MS. Not all hyaluronic acid dermal fillers are equal. Cosmetic Dermatology. 2007;20(11):724–729.

Kablik J, Monheit GD, Yu L, et al. Comparative physical properties of hyaluronic acid dermal fillers. Derm Surg. 2009;(35 Suppl 1):302–312.

Monheit GD, Coleman KM. Hyaluronic acid fillers. Dermatol Ther. 2006;19(3):141–150.

Weinkle SH, Bank DE, Boyd CM, et al. A multi-center, double-blind, randomized controlled study of the safety and effectiveness of Juvederm injectable gel with and without lidocaine. J Cosmet Dermatol. 2009;8(3):205–210.

## Calcium Hydroxylapatite Dermal Fillers

Berlin AL, Hussain M, Goldberg DJ. Calcium hydroxylapatite filler for facial rejuvenation: a histologic and immunohistochemical analysis. Dermatol Surg. 2008;34(Suppl):S64–S67.

Busso M, Voigts R. An investigation of changes in physical properties of injectable calcium hydroxylapatite in a carrier gel when mixed with lidocaine and with lidocaine/epinephrine. Dermatol Surg. 2008;34(Suppl 1):S16–S23.

Carruthers A, Liebeskind M, Carruthers J, et al. Radiographic and computed tomographic studies of calcium hydroxylapatite for treatment of HIV-associated facial lipoatrophy and correction of nasolabial folds. Dermatol Surg. 2008;34(Suppl 1):S78–S84.

Jansen DA, Graivier MH. Evaluation of a calcium hydroxylapatite-based implant (Radiesse) for facial soft-tissue augmentation. Plast Reconstr Surg. 2006;118(3 Suppl):22S–30S.

Marmur E, Green L, Busso M. Controlled, randomized study of pain levels in subjects treated with calcium hydroxylapatite premixed with lidocaine for correction of nasolabial folds. Dermatol Surg. 2010;36(3):309–315.

## Anesthesia

Foley K, Pianalto D. Facial Anesthesia. Emerg Med. 2005;37(6):30–34.

Henning JS, Firoz BF. The use of a cooling device as an analgesic before injectable local anesthesia in the pediatric population. Dermatol Surg. 2010;36(4):520–523.

Kawesk S. Topical anesthetic creams [Safety and Efficacy Report]. Plast Reconstr Surg. 2008;121(6):2161–2165.

Lee MS. Topical triple-anesthetic gel compared with 3 topical anesthetics. Cosmetic Dermatology. 2003;26(61);35–38.

Niamtu J, III. Simple technique for lip and nasolabial fold anesthesia for injectable fillers. Dermatol Surg. 2005;31(10):1330–1332.

Salam G, et al. Regional anesthesia for office procedures: Part 1. Head and neck surgeries. Am Fam Phys. 2004;69(3):585–590.

Small R. Anesthesia for Cosmetic Procedures. In: Usatine R, Pfenninger J, Stuhlberg D, Small R, eds. Dermatologic and Cosmetic Procedures in Office Practice. Philadelphia, PA: Elsevier; 2011;241–247.

Smith KC. Ice anesthesia for injection of dermal fillers. Dermatol Surg. 2010;36:812–814.

Weiss RA, Lavin PT. Reduction of pain and anxiety prior to botulinum toxin injections with a new topical anesthetic method. Ophthal Plast Reconstr Surg. 2009;25(3):173–177.

## Storing and Reusing Dermal Fillers

Safo PK, Wahlgren C, Obagi S. Safety of Storing and Reusing Hyaluronic Acid Fillers: A Retrospective Chart Review. Cosmet Dermatol. 2011;24:22–27.

## Dermal Filler Treatment Areas

### Nasolabial Folds

Alam M, Yoo SS. Technique for calcium hydroxylapatite injection for correction of nasolabial fold depressions. J Am Acad Dermatol. 2007;56(2):285–289.

Graivier MH. Correcting nasolabial folds. Cosmetic Surg Times. 2006;1–8.

Heden P, Fagrell D, Jernbeck J, et al. Injection of stabilized hyaluronic acid-based gel of non-animal origin for the correction of nasolabial folds: comparison with and without lidocaine. Dermatol Surg. 2010;36:775–781.

Lupo MP, Smith SR, Thomas JA, et al. Effectiveness of Juvederm Ultra Plus dermal filler in the treatment of severe nasolabial folds. Plast Reconstr Surg. 2008;121(1):289–297.

Marmur ES, Taylor SC, Grimes PE, et al. Six-month safety results of calcium hydroxylapatite for treatment of nasolabial folds in Fitzpatrick skin types IV to VI. Dermatol Surg. 2009;35(Suppl 2):1641–1645.

Moers-Carpi M, Vogt S, Santos BM, et al. A multicenter, randomized trial comparing calcium hydroxylapatite to two hyaluronic acids for treatment of nasolabial folds. Dermatol Surg. 33(Suppl 2):S144–S151.

Narins RS, Brandt FS, Leyden J, et al. A randomized, double-blind, multicenter comparison of the efficacy and tolerability of Restylane versus Zyplast for the correction of nasolabial folds. Dermatol Surg. 2003;29(6):588–595.

Smith SR, Busso M, McClaren M, et al. A randomized, bilateral, prospective comparison of calcium hydroxylapatite microspheres versus human-based collagen for the correction of nasolabial folds. Dermatol Surg. 2007;33(Suppl 2):S112–S121.

Weiss RA, Bank D, Brandt FS. Randomized, double-blind, split-face study of small-gel-particle hyaluronic acid with and without lidocaine during correction of nasolabial folds. Dermatol Surg. 2010;36:750–759.

## Lip Augmentation

Ali MJ, Ende K, Maas CS. Perioral rejuvenation and lip augmentation. Facial Plast Surg Clin North Am. 2007;15(4):491–500, vii.

Lanigan S. An observational study of a 24 mg/mL hyaluronic acid with pre-incorporated lidocaine for lip definition and enhancement. J Cosmet Dermatol. 2011;10(1):11–14.

Solish N, Swift A. An open-label, pilot study to assess the effectiveness and safety of hyaluronic acid gel in the restoration of soft tissue fullness of the lips. J Drugs Dermatol. 2011;10(2):145–149.

## Other Facial Areas

Belmontesi M, Grover R, Verpaele A. Transdermal injection of Restylane SubQ for aesthetic contouring of the cheeks, chin, and mandible. Aesthet Surg J. 2006;26(1S):S28–S34.

Busso M, Karlsburg PL. Cheek augmentation and rejuvenation using injectable calcium hydroxylapatite (radiesse). Cosmetic Dermatology. 2006;19(9):583–588.

Lowe NJ, Grover R. Injectable hyaluronic acid implant for malar and mental enhancement. Dermatol Surg. 2006;32(7):881–885.

Sclafani AP, Kwak E. Alternative management of the aging jawline and neck. Facial Plast Surg. 2005;21(1):47–54.

Verpaele A, Strand A. Restylane SubQ, a non-animal stabilized hyaluronic acid gel for soft tissue augmentation of the mid- and lower face. Aesthet Surg J. 2006;26(1S):S10–S17.

Weinkle S. Injection techniques for revolumization of the perioral region with hyaluronic acid. J Drugs Dermatol. 2010;9(4):367–371.

## Combining Aesthetic Treatments

Carruthers A, Carruthers J, Monheit GD, et al. Multicenter, randomized, parallel-group study of the safety and effectiveness of onabotulinumtoxinA and hyaluronic acid dermal fillers (24-mg/ml smooth, cohesive gel) alone and in combination for lower facial rejuvenation. Dermatol Surg. 2010;36(Suppl 4):2121–2134.

Carruthers J, Carruthers A, Maberley D. Deep resting glabellar rhytides respond to BTX-A and Hylan B. Derm Surg. 2003;29(5):539–544.

Carruthers JD, Carruthers A. A prospective, randomized, parallel group study analyzing the effect of BTX-A (Botox) and nonanimal sourced hyaluronic acid (NASHA, Restylane) in combination compared with NASHA (Restylane) alone in severe glabellar rhytides in adult female subjects: treatment of severe glabellar rhytides with a hyaluronic acid derivative compared with the derivative and BTX-A. Dermatol Surg. 2003;29(8):802–809.

Carruthers JD, Glogau RG, Blitzer A. Advances in facial rejuvenation: botulinum toxin type a, hyaluronic acid dermal fillers, and combination therapies–consensus recommendations. Plast Reconstr Surg. 2008;121(5 Suppl):5S–30S.

Coleman KR, Carruthers J. Combination therapy with BOTOX and fillers: the new rejuvnation paradigm. Dermatol Ther. 2006;19(3):177–188.

Godin MS, Majmundar MV, Chrzanowski DS, et al. Use of radiesse in combination with restylane for facial augmentation. Arch Facial Plast Surg. 2006;8(2)92–97.

Maas CS. Botulinum neurotoxins and injectable fillers: minimally invasive management of the aging upper face. Facial Plast Surg Clin North Am. 2006;14(3):241–245.

Small R, Hoang D. Combining Cosmetic Treatments. In: Usatine R, Pfenninger J, Stuhlberg D, Small R, eds. Dermatologic and Cosmetic Procedures in Office Practice. Philadelphia, PA. Elsevier. 2011;377–382.

## Complications Dermal Fillers

Bachmann F, Erdmann R, Hartmann V, et al. The spectrum of adverse reactions after treatment with injectable fillers in the glabellar region: results from the Injectable Filler Safety Study. Dermatol Surg. 2009;35(Suppl 2):1629–1634.

Baumann LS, Romanelli P, Marangoni O, et al. Keratoacanthomas as complication of dermal filler injections. Cosmetic Dermatology. 2007;20(7):450–452.

Brody HJ. Use of hyaluronidase in the treatment of granulomatous hyaluronic acid reactions or unwanted hyaluronic acid misplacement. Dermatol Surg. 2005;31(8 Pt 1):893–897.

Cassuto D, Marangoni O, De SG, et al. Advanced laser techniques for filler-induced complications. Dermatol Surg. 2009;35(Suppl 2):1689–1695.

Chabra I, Obagi S. Severe site reaction after injecting hyaluronic acid-based soft tissue filler. Cosmetic Dermatology. 2011;24(1):14–21.

Cohen JL. Understanding, avoiding, and managing dermal filler complications. Dermatol Surg. 2008;34(Suppl 1): S92–S99.

Coleman KR, Carruthers J. Combination therapy with BOTOX and fillers: the new rejuvenation paradigm. Dermatol Ther. 2006;19(3):177–188.

Cox SE. Clinical experience with filler complications. Dermatol Surg. 2009;35:1661–1666.

DeLorenzi C, Weinberg M, Solish N, et al. The long-term efficacy and safety of a subcutaneously injected large-particle stabilized hyaluronic acid-based gel of nonanimal origin in esthetic facial contouring. Dermatol Surg. 2009;35(Suppl 1):313–321.

Geisler D, Shumer S, Elson M. Delayed hypersensitivity reaction to restylane. Cosmetic Dermatology. 2007;20(12):784–786.

Gladstone HB, Cohen JL. Adverse effects when injecting facial fillers. Semin Cutan Med Surg. 2007;26(1):34–39.

Glogau RG, Kane MA. Effect of injection techniques on the rate of local adverse events in patients implanted with nonanimal hyaluronic acid gel dermal fillers. Dermatol Surg. 2008;34(Suppl 1):S105–S109.

Goldman MP. Superficial nodularity of hydroxylapatite filler to fill the infraorbital hollow. Dermatol Surg. 2010;36:822–824.

Grunebaum LD, Allemann IB, Dayan S, et al. The risk of alar necrosis associated with dermal filler injection. Dermatol Surg. 2009;35:1635–1640.

Hirsch RJ, Cohen JL, Carruthers JD. Successful management of an unusual presentation of impending necrosis following a hyaluronic acid injection embolus and a proposed algorithm for management with hyaluronidase. Dermatol Surg. 2007;33(3):357–360.

Hirsch RJ, Narurkar V, Carruthers J. Management of injected hyaluronic acid induced Tyndall effects. Lasers Surg Med. 2006;38(3):202–204.

Junkins-Hopkins JM. Filler complications. J Am Acad Dermatol. 2010;63(4):703–705.

Lee A, Grummer SE, Kriegel D, et al. Hyaluronidase. Dermatol Surg. 2010;36(7):1071–1077.

Lowe NJ, Maxwell CA, Patnaik R. Adverse reactions to dermal fillers: review. Dermatol Surg. 2005;31 (11 Pt 2):1616–1625.

Narins RS, Coleman WP, III, Glogau RG. Recommendations and treatment options for nodules and other filler complications. Dermatol Surg. 2009;35(Suppl 2):1667–1671.

Narins RS, Jewell M, Rubin M, et al. Clinical conference: management of rare events following dermal fillers-Focal necrosis and angry red bumps. Dermatol Surg. 2006;32(3):426–434.

Rohrich RJ, Monheit G, Nguyen AT, et al. Soft-tissue filler complications: the important role of biofilms. Plast Reconstr Surg. 2010;125(4):1250–1256.

Requena L, Requena C, Christensen L, et al. Adverse reactions to injectable soft tissue fillers. J Am Acad Dermatol. 2011;64(1):1–34.

Schanz S, Schippert W, Ulmer A, et al. Arterial embolization caused by injection of hyaluronic acid (Restylane). Brit J Dermatol. 2002;146(5):928–929.

Sclafani AP, Fagien S. Treatment of injectable soft tissue filler complications. Dermatol Surg. 2009;35 (Suppl 2):1672–1680.

Sperling B, Bachmann F, Hartmann V, et al. The current state of treatment of adverse reactions to injectable fillers. Dermatol Surg. 2010;36(Suppl 3):1895–1904.

Van DS, Hays GP, Caglia AE, et al. Severe acute local reactions to a hyaluronic acid-derived dermal filler. J Clin Aesthet Dermatol. 2010;3(5):32–35.

Vartanian AJ, Frankel AS, Rubin MG. Injected hyaluronidase reduces restylane-mediated cutaneous augmentation. Arch Facial Plast Surg. 2005;7(4):231–237.

Zielke H, Wolber L, Wiest L, et al. Risk profiles of different injectable fillers: results from the Injectable Filler Safety Study (IFS Study). Dermatol Surg. 2008;34(3):326–335.

## Complications Anesthesia

Hahn IH, Hoffman RS, Nelson LS. EMLA-induced methemoglobinemia and systemic topical anesthetic toxicity. J Emerg Med. 2004;26(1):85–88.

Kaweski S. Topical anesthetic creams. Plast Reconstr Surg. 2008;121(6):2161–2165.

Lacy CF, Armstrong LL, Goldman MP, et al. Drug Information Handbook. 20th ed. Hudson: Lexicomp Inc, 2011.

Marra DE, Yip D, Fincher EF, et al. Systemic toxicity from topically applied lidocaine in conjunction with fractional photothermolysis. Arch Dermatol. 142(8):1024–1026, 2006.

Physicians Desk Reference. 65th ed. Montvale, NJ. Thompson PDR. 2011.

Touma S, Jackson JB. Lidocaine and prilocaine toxicity in a patient receiving treatment for molusca contagiosa. J Am Acad Dermatol. 2001;44(2 suppl):399–400.

Note: Page numbers followed by f and t denotes figure and table respectively.